P9-DVH-568

NEW YOU
BOOT CAMP

' Loss: 13lbs. A dress size. 3½ inches from the waist. 1½ inches from each thigh. 1½ inches from the hips. 1 inch from each arm. Thirteen Pounds! This is better than liposuction! It's a dress size. I am a 12 again. I LOVE being a soldier.'

Mail on Sunday Sharon Marshall,
New You Boot Camp Breacon Beacons

We would like to dedicate this book to all of our clients who have already found their NEW YOU since starting their journey with us, and to all of you who are just about to start your journey to the NEW YOU. Enjoy the journey, and enjoy the NEW YOU.

First published in the United Kingdom in 2010 by Collins & Brown
10 Southcombe Street
London
W14 0RA

An imprint of Anova Books Company Ltd

Copyright © Collins & Brown 2010

Text copyright © Sunny Moran & Jacqui Cleaver/Collins & Brown 2010

Distributed in the United States and Canada by Sterling Publishing Co, 387 Park Avenue South, New York, NY 10016, USA

ISBN 978-1-84340-561-0

A CIP catalogue for this book is available from the British Library.

10 9 8 7 6 5 4 3 2 1

Reproduction by Rival Colour UK Ltd

Printed and bound by Mondadori, Cles, Italy

This book can be ordered direct from the publisher at www.anovabooks.com

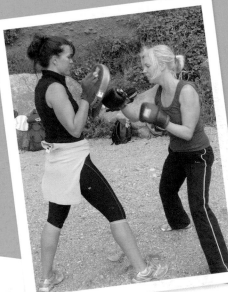

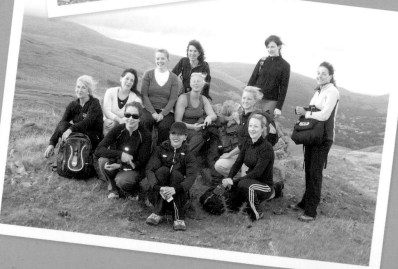

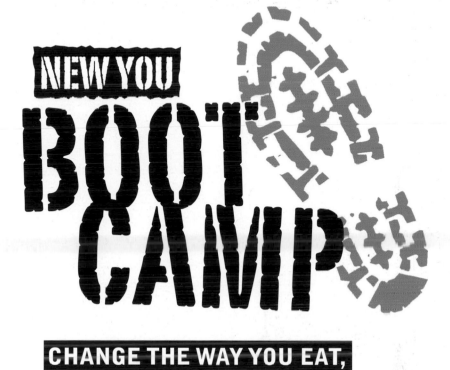

NEW YOU
BOOT CAMP

CHANGE THE WAY YOU EAT,
THINK AND EXERCISE FOR LIFE

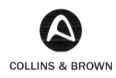

COLLINS & BROWN

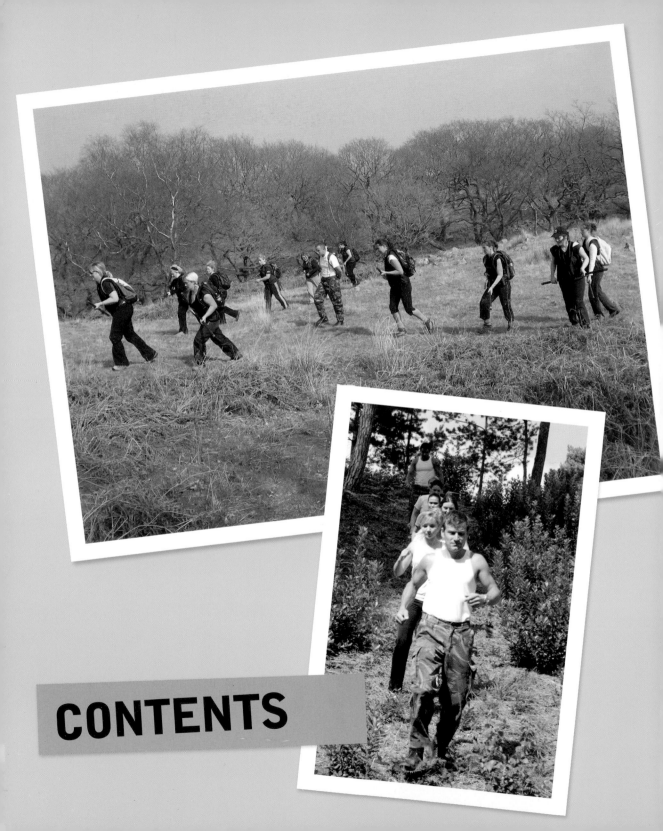

CONTENTS

Introduction 6

8   **New You Boot Camp – Behind the Story**
10 **Why New You Boot Camp Works**
12 **How To Use This Book**
14 **My Personal Commitment**

Boot Camp Mindset 16

18 **Setting Goals**
20 **My Goals**
22 **Make It Happen!**
24 **Believe in Yourself**
26 **New You Boot Camp Diary**
28 **Before You Begin**
30 **Success Story**

Training 32

34 **Why Exercise?**
36 **Make Time to Train**
38 **Get the Gear**
40 **Starting Point**
44 **The Two-Week Drop-a-Dress-Size Plan**
46 **Warm Ups**
50 **The Cardio Workouts**
54 **The Strength Workouts**
66 **What Next?**
80 **Success Stories**

Nutrition 82

84   **The New You Boot Camp Four-Step Plan**
86   **How Does it Work?**
88   **Choose Your Food**
92   **New You Boot Camp 10 Commandments**
94   **Eating Fat**
96   **New You Boot Camp and Alcohol**
98   **Dispelling Diet Myths**
100 **New You Boot Camp Two-Week Menu Plan**
104 **Recipes**
134 **Success Stories**

Life After New You Boot Camp 136

138 **New You Forever**
140 **New You Everyday Exercise**
146 **Get Your Family and Friends Active**
148 **Food For Special Occasions**
150 **Golden Rules for Eating Out**
152 **Success Stories**
154 **New You Boot Camp Back Up Forum**

156 **Index**
158 **Picture credits**
159 **Author acknowledgements**

Introduction

Welcome to New You Boot Camp and congratulations on taking your first step towards the New You. There are plenty of fitness camps and health regimes that promise to help you lose weight and stay in shape, but no other fitness boot camp or health spa is as successful as we are. Our results speak for themselves.

Over the course of the fifty-plus boot camps that New You Boot Camp have held we have helped clients lose a staggering 714 stone and 9,115 inches. And now, for the first time, you don't need to come to New You Boot Camp to share in this success. We're going to share our secrets with you right here, right now!

We chose the name 'New You' for our boot camps because we really believe we can show you how to change the habits that are holding you back and become a new person. The very best person you can be. Reading this book and following our advice is your first step on the path to discovering a New You. We won't just help you lose weight, but will build your confidence so nothing can hold you back. Your self-esteem will grow by a mile and every part of your life will improve.

'Diet' is a word that we don't like to use at New You Boot Camp. Believe us, we've tried every diet under the sun and we know what works and what's a waste of time. In this book we go back to basics and teach you how to eat well. The good news is that starving yourself or following the latest crazy diet are off the menu! New You Boot Camp is a lifestyle – we don't ask you to count calories, carbohydrates or points, nor do we ask you to make drinks with strange ingredients you've never heard of, or skip meals. If you follow our simple Boot Camp rules you'll eat three meals a day plus two snacks and learn how to make sensible food choices that will help you achieve your weight loss goals no matter how busy you are! There's a two-week menu plan to start you off, or skip straight to our Four-Step Plan, a simple system you can use every day to choose foods that will give you energy and keep you trim day in and day out.

We all know that healthy eating works best when combined with exercise, so we've hooked the simple two-week eating plan up with a two-week plan to boost your activity levels. Our exercises have been specially developed by world-class trainers and include cardiovascular, fat-burning and PT sessions that promise you amazing results. So if you feel as though you're in a rut, can't seem to change your habits and need a kick-start, start the New You Boot Camp programme today. We know you'll find the self-confidence and motivational boost you deserve. Our promise to YOU is that when you follow the New You Boot Camp two-week nutrition and exercise plan, you'll not only lose weight and feel fighting fit, you'll know that you can do and achieve anything if you put your mind to it!

Your best body ever, bags of energy and unshakeable self-belief: stick to our rules and you WILL have them all, we promise!

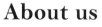

About us

New You Boot Camp was founded by us: Sunny and Jacqui, and we'd like to tell you how it came about. We were friends at college but pursued separate careers in different parts of the world. Over the years we both tried every diet under the sun: from Atkins to a popcorn and Diet Coke one! We'd been a teeny size 8 and a generous size 18, with our weight yo-yoing up and down as we tried one fad after another. By our late twenties it was finally sinking in that there are no short cuts when it comes to losing weight. To get results something had to change. We'd both reached that same point in our lives when we got together to catch up over a coffee.

As we chatted about our weight problems, the idea that became New You Boot Camp was born. Why shouldn't we use our passion for diet and fitness to help not just ourselves, but others too? We'd heard about American boot camps and liked the idea of strict discipline and a back-to-basics approach. We tried some of the weight-loss camps on offer at the time and found that lots of them were great while they lasted, but after the week was over it was just too easy to slip back into old habits. Fundamentally nothing changed.

Lots of diets work: we'd proved that. But why don't they last? We discovered the truth when we finally stopped looking for what was wrong with the diets and started looking at ourselves. The truth we discovered is that you can only change your body if you start by changing your mind. You have to stop making excuses and start believing in yourself.

We're not saying it isn't hard work. It's because it is hard work that you have to change the way you think. Losing weight requires effort, it requires determination and it demands that you devote some time to looking after yourself. And you can only do that if you believe that you are worth it and that you will stick with it and achieve your goals. At New You Boot Camp we hear the same stories every time: our clients don't have time to exercise; they're too exhausted to cook food from scratch; when are they supposed to find the time to plan their menu and shop properly? We don't give them easy answers. They have to accept that they must find the time to do those things. They have to shift their priorities to include themselves. We know it's not easy if you've spent a lifetime looking after other people or thinking you're just not worth the effort because you always fail anyway, so we concentrate on helping you believe in yourself.

We don't believe in setting you up to fail either. We're both normal girls; we like to party and we have our off days like everyone else. We've created a programme that allows for that and even encourages it, so you can carry on losing weight and feeling good about yourself and still have a life!

New You Boot Camp was a leap of faith for us. We gave up well-paid jobs because we believed we could do something more worthwhile. We trusted that we wouldn't fail, and we haven't. At every New You Boot Camp we see moving transformations with clients leaving us not only fitter but also with a new-found sense of confidence and self-belief. And now we want to pass on that self-belief to you, because that's all it takes to make anything possible. Just as we've made friends with our clients at New You Boot Camp and are there to support them we want to be there to support you.

We've also lost three stone each: and finally managed to keep it off! If we can do it so can you!

Jacqui Weaver and Sunny Moran

Founders of New You Boot Camp

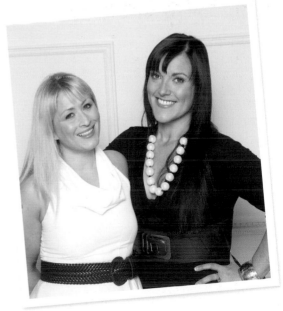

Why New You Boot Camp Works

The bookshops are full of diet books, so what's so great about this one? We've learned the hard way that quick fixes don't work, so New You Boot Camp is different. It works because:

- There are no gimmicks, just easy-to-follow straightforward advice so you can make the right choices to keep you healthy every day.

- It's practical and flexible so you'll be able to fit it into your everyday life.

- It's designed for real people like you and me who want to have a life!

- After the initial two-week Drop-a-Dress-Size plan, our simple diet and exercise guidelines can be followed for life, so you won't slip back into your old habits. Don't just put the book down when you've done your two-week stint. Keep it close by to stay on track for good.

- It's healthy and safe. The only damage this book can inflict is paper cuts!

- We're normal girls who like to party just the same as you, and we know that sometimes life gets in the way of good intentions, so don't worry if you go off the rails once in a while. We all have bad days. Just keep going!

- This book works *with* your mind and body, not against it.

- You don't have to starve yourself like on some crazy diets. You get to eat, have a life, lose weight and have plenty of energy to enjoy yourself.

- It's designed to be fun and to get results fast. The exercises combine a tough strength training workout with challenging cardio moves to maximize your fat burning and help you get great results fast.

- It comes with an inbuilt support network: you can find others who are going through the same experience on our New You Boot Camp forum.

We promise that if you follow this plan you'll see results in as little as two weeks. Stick at it and soon you'll discover a New You. Healthy eating and exercise will be as much a part of your life as breathing and you can banish your body blues forever and face life with renewed energy and confidence.

"What other New You Boot Campers have said"

I want to congratulate you on developing a great product; the programme docs deliver. I have felt calm and focused since completing New You Boot Camp and with a new sense of 'can do' ... I have also got my old mountain bike out, bought proper running shoes and had gait assessment to continue the 'new' skills long forgotten.

Diana Terry

After losing 8lbs at New You Boot Camp I lost a further 6lbs last week, so feeling much better for being a stone lighter. I'm being very virtuous but have some 'challenges' ahead including hen weekends and weddings so might have to adopt the 80/20 rule those weekends!

Kelly Radley

New You Boot Camp was a fantastic journey for me and I have learnt lots that I can add to my current routine. My goal is to now maintain what I have achieved, and to build myself up to get fitter, faster and stronger.
In the words of Arnie... 'I'll be back!'

Dawn Kneen

How To Use This Book

Follow these ten simple steps to reveal the New You. Not just for two weeks, but for the rest of your life.

1 Start today. The first thing we want you to do is read the book through. Then don't just put it down and forget about it. Take ownership of your life and the changes you want to make.

2 Set your goals. Read the Boot Camp Mindset section on page 17 to help you pin down what you want to achieve. There's space in that section to write down your goals, or if you prefer you can get started right away on your New You Boot Camp diary (see page 26) and write your goals at the beginning of that.

3 Look at the Personal Commitment on page 14 and sign and date it. This is a really important part of the New You Boot Camp process. It's your promise to yourself that you'll do what it takes to achieve your goals. No excuses. Look back at this page whenever your commitment is flagging so you never forget why you started. Stick your 'before' picture here or in your diary and look forward to the delicious 'after' photo to come!

Sticking to a diet and exercise plan for two weeks might sound gruelling, but you'll get far more out of it than losing a few pounds. You'll find reserves of discipline you never knew you had and discover that you're capable of much more than you ever imagined.

4 Complete the self-assessment tests (see page 40) to check your fitness levels today. If you haven't already done it, start a diary to record your results and write down what happens as you begin to exercise and follow the nutrition plan. If you keep track of how you're doing you'll soon be able to see the results of all your hard work in black and white.

5 Plan your week ahead so that you can start our two-week Drop-a-Dress-Size plan. If you're struggling to find the time to exercise, get up earlier like our clients at New You Boot Camp. Your goals are important so take the time to achieve them.

6 Check out the nutrition section (see page 83) and work out what you'll be eating for the next two weeks. You can choose to follow our two-week menu plan to get you started, or dive straight into the New You Boot Camp Four-Step Plan. Both will kick-start you into a new way of eating that is healthy, nutritious and so simple that you'll have no problems staying trim for good.

7 Ditch the junk from your kitchen cupboards and fill them with the healthy foods you're going to be enjoying from now on. See page 133 for top tips on saintly snacks you can enjoy guilt-free.

8 If you feel your resolve beginning to crumble, flip through the book to check out our motivational tips. The Boot Camp Mindset section (see page 17) has our top techniques to keep you on track.

9 Stay in touch with your fellow New You Boot Campers using our online forum (see page 154). Sharing what you're going through with others who are in the same boat makes any problems seem far less daunting.

10 Once you've completed the two-week plan, keep up the good work with the At Home circuits and the Life After New You Boot Camp section. The benefits of New You Boot Camp will go on long after you have read this book. This is the beginning of the New You.

MY PERSONAL COMMITMENT

Congratulations! Taking the first step to the New You will be one of the best decisions of your life. You're on your way to a new, healthier, better lifestyle.

When you've read through the book, and understand what you're letting yourself in for, sign and date this Personal Commitment and refer back to it regularly to check that you're sticking to the promises you've made to yourself.

1 I commit to the New You Boot Camp Fitness Programme, starting with the two-week fitness plan. After I've finished the two-week plan I will maintain my fitness levels by using the circuit training plans to train for 40 minutes four or five times every week.

2 I commit to following the simple New You Boot Camp nutrition and eating plan and to staying within the rules. Consistency and commitment are the key to achieving results.

3 I commit to setting SMARTER goals and achieving them.

4 I commit to eating every three hours and sticking to five smaller meals or three meals and two snacks each day. I will not skip meals.

5 I will stick strictly to the plan for two weeks, and then follow the 80:20 rule, which states that if I stick to the rules 80% of the time I can treat myself 20% of the time, or give myself one day off a week, within the nutrition rules.

6 I commit to drinking at least 2–3 litres (3½–5 pints) of water a day, despite the toilet breaks!

7 I commit to getting my beauty sleep – eight hours a night, so I wake up looking refreshed and knowing I'll function more efficiently. Sleep is my recovery time.

8 I commit to believing in myself and knowing that I deserve the health and wellbeing my new lifestyle will bring.

I (enter name) ....
promise to follow this personal commitment to the best of my ability.

Signed: .... Date: ....

BEFORE & AFTER
Photos

Add a photo of yourself either on this page or in your New You Boot Camp diary before you begin the programme. Update the 'after' photo at regular intervals and soon you'll see a fit and foxy new you emerge.

BEFORE

AFTER

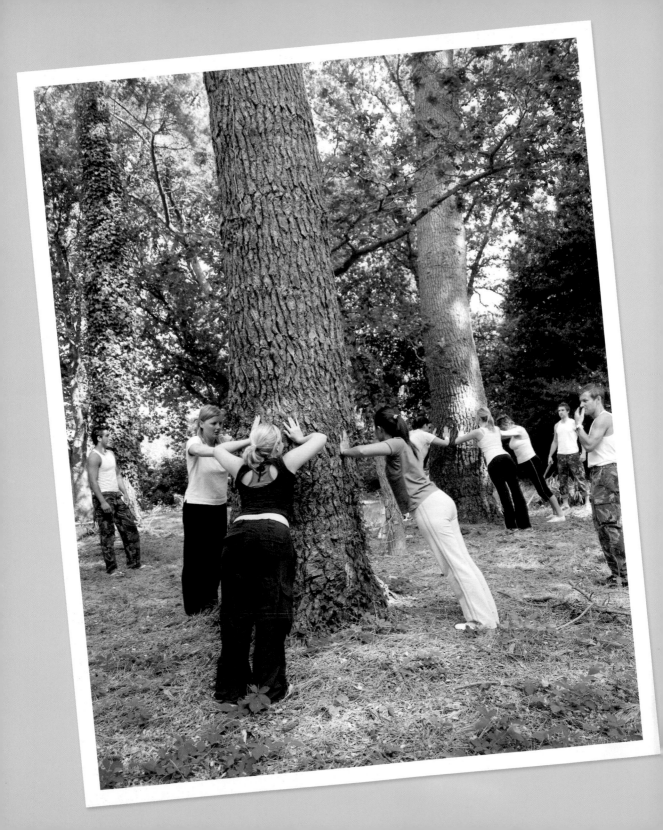

Boot Camp Mindset

We've been on plenty of diets and know how hard it is to stay on track when the going gets tough. In this section we're going to share our best-kept trade secrets with you: the motivational techniques that will make sure you see *this* programme through no matter how many others you've thrown away in disgust. What you eat and the exercise you do are important to the New You programme, but not as vital as how you think. We're going to teach you how to set achievable goals for yourself, put yourself in the best frame of mind to achieve those goals, and how to pick yourself up, dust yourself off and start all over again when things don't quite go to plan. Most importantly, we'll teach you to believe that you can achieve anything if you put your mind to it.

My Goals

Now you know the theory it's time to put it into practice. We want you to set yourself three goals: one for one month's time, one for three months' time and one for the longer term. Follow the SMARTER rules we showed you on page 18 and don't forget to write down your reward. You can write them here or in your New You Boot Camp diary and we think it's a great idea to copy them out and pin them up somewhere you'll see them every day. The more you see them, the more real they will become.

Believe in yourself. The more often you tell yourself 'I can and I will', the more likely it is to be true. If you allow yourself to think negatively you'll undermine your confidence and sabotage your efforts to reach your goals.

One-month SMARTER goal

Think about where you want to be in one month. Our two-week Drop-a-Dress-Size plan will get you off to a flying start, so be ambitious, but not unrealistic. This could mean doing a 5km (3-mile) fun run (yes, you can!) or simply lifting your mood and self-esteem by sticking to your fitness plan. Think of a (non-edible) reward such as a new CD, a pedicure or a movie. When you reach your goal, make sure you give yourself the reward.

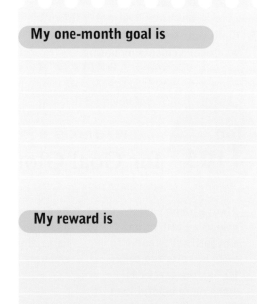

My one-month goal is

My reward is

Three-month goal

Decide where you want to be in three months' time and make the reward just a bit bigger. So, you might decide you're going to lose a certain amount of weight or improve your fitness levels so that you can run for the bus without getting breathless. Your reward could be buying a pair of shoes, getting a day's worth of beauty treatments at the salon or going away for a special weekend.

Long-term goal

Figure out what you ultimately want to achieve and by when you (realistically) think you can do it. You might want to reach a certain dress size and get into your favourite jeans or bikini. Set up a holiday for that date or find another way to celebrate your achievement. Give yourself a little leeway here. Don't cancel a trip or punish yourself if you are 3lbs off. The point is to look forward to something.

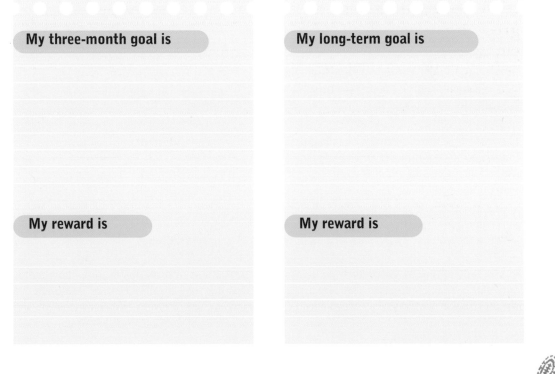

My three-month goal is

My reward is

My long-term goal is

My reward is

Make It Happen!

Are you looking forward to achieving your New You Boot Camp goals? Do you believe that you can do it? If you have a little wobble now and then and start to lose faith, don't worry – we've all been there. Now we're going to share with you some tricks we use to keep our campers focused and help them to make their dreams a reality.

When you start the New You Boot Camp programme you're likely to be focusing on the exercises and eating plan. Of course these are the core of the programme and are really important, but we also want to teach you how to use your mind as well as your body to achieve your goals. Your ability to do anything in life depends on how you control your thoughts, whether you're walking, swimming, reading a book, eating or exercising. Ultimately, if you can communicate more effectively not only with others, but, most importantly, with yourself then your goals will be far more achievable. Your mind holds the key to your new body.

The first trick up our sleeve is visualization. There's nothing gimmicky or New-Agey about this, it's just an extension of something we all do all the time. We're simply going to ask you to imagine how you're going to look, think, feel and act once you've achieved your goals. Simple as that.

So how's that going to help? Well, let's start with a simple exercise to show you just what a powerful effect your mind can have on your body:

> Sit down, close your eyes and imagine you've been out all day and you're extremely thirsty. Visualize yourself going to your fridge, opening the door, reaching in and picking up the biggest yellow lemon you can find. Now go to a drawer and pick up a sharp knife and cut the lemon into big thick segments. Smell the beautiful citrus smell and now lift one half to your mouth and bite into it, allowing all the fresh citrus juices to swirl in your mouth.

Do you feel as though you can taste the lemon? Did your mouth water just at the thought of those bitter juices flowing? This is a very simple example, and we're not suggesting for one moment that you can eat what you like and ignore the exercise plan as long as you 'think thin', but it does illustrate the very powerful effect that your mind can have on your body. Now we'd like you to take that knowledge and use it to help you create your own ideal future.

This technique sounds simple, but don't be deceived. It's an incredibly powerful way of focusing your mind and harnessing your inner resources to achieve success.

New You Visualization

First find a quiet place where you know you won't be disturbed. Sit or lie down, then close your eyes and breathe deeply for a few minutes, in through your nose and out through your mouth.

Now focus your mind on the goals you want to achieve in the next year.

Imagine how it feels to accomplish your goals. How do you look? How are you acting? What are the emotions that come to you? Make sure you don't just SEE this in your visualization: you must actually FEEL it. It's important that you visualize from the first person and not as an outsider looking in. You must BE you.

Be sure to visualize a real-life movie, not a photo or static screen. Why don't you create a whole story in your head with you in the role of leading lady or hero? This will help you to act and feel the part. Have you ever heard the term 'Living The Dream'? Well, this is what this is about. The movie WILL become a reality, but only if you stay focused and constantly tune in to your movie. Any time you feel your will power wavering, take five, close your eyes and run your own private show.

Believe In Yourself

If you're reading this book then you're already at a turning point in your life. Whatever has brought you to this point, whether it's low confidence, an unhealthy lifestyle, weight gain or a mixture of all these reasons, you're ready to change. Now. And it's not just your body that you're going to change. It's the way you think too.

If you're ever going to accomplish your goals you must start from a point where you believe two fundamental things:

- That you are capable of changing

- That you deserve to change

So many of us go through life beating ourselves up over one thing or another. Telling ourselves that we're not good enough, that we're not able to change or, more insidiously, that we somehow don't deserve the life we imagine our slimmer or fitter friends are leading. Negative thinking like that attracts a negative reality and sabotages your efforts to change. We're here to tell you that it needs to stop right here and right now. We know that if you change your thought processes then you can and will change your reality.

We have two strategies to beat the kind of negative thinking that can wreck your best efforts to stick to the programme. The first is positive action. Start the programme.

Buy the foods. Make time for the exercise programme, however difficult it seems. If you're busy exercising, cooking healthy food and filling in your New You Boot Camp diary, then you'll have less time to dwell on negative thoughts.

The second is positive thinking. Crowd out the negative thoughts with positive ones. Every time you catch yourself slipping into your old destructive mindset, turn those thoughts around. If you find yourself thinking you're lazy, remind yourself of all the effort you've made. If you think breaking the nutrition rules won't matter because you never lose any weight anyway, then remind yourself you have lost weight and will lose more. See the box opposite for some other ways to turn those negative thoughts on their head and fill your mind with something healthier and more productive.

We should warn you that you might feel uncomfortable doing this at first. You might feel a bit of a fraud. You might simply find it hard to believe that it can possibly make any difference. If you've spent a large part of your life convincing yourself that you're useless, unattractive and don't deserve a better life, then that's what you'll believe in your heart. But trust us. You might not believe what you're telling yourself, but persevere. If your head insists then your heart will soon have no choice but to believe and success *will* follow.

Focus on the Positive

Most people are very self-critical. Try to be your own biggest fan. Wake up every day and give yourself a cheer! Think positively about who you are and what you've achieved and will achieve in the future. Concentrate on the parts of yourself that you love (yes, you will find some if you try hard enough: see our next point below). Say to yourself, 'I look great in this dress' or 'I'm having a good hair day'. This doesn't mean that you should be arrogant or conceited, as neither of these are very attractive characteristics, but confidence and self-appreciation most definitely are.

How many of you concentrate on areas of your body you don't like? Most of you would probably answer 'yes' to this question as that's the normal reaction. Instead of concentrating on the negatives, find the part of you that you love. Everyone has some positive quality. It can be anything from the colour of your eyes to your clear skin or healthy-looking hair.

We'll say it again: how you think is just as important as what you eat and your exercise plan. You have to believe in yourself and know that you are fabulous. Keep repeating to yourself, 'I deserve this new life – I am worth it!' If you expect to succeed, you will.

New You Boot Camp *Diary*

We'd like to introduce you to your new best friend – your New You Boot Camp diary. You can carry on confiding in your girlfriends if you like, but only after you've written everything down in your diary. Soon it will hold the key that unlocks your success.

Buy yourself a notebook or diary or set up a log book on your computer that you can update daily. Write down your Personal Commitment (see page 14), your goals and the results of the fitness assessments on pages 40-43. If you want to, you can put your 'before' photo in your diary as well. Don't forget to leave space for that stunning 'after' shot that's coming soon!

Top Tip

Find a way of keeping a diary that suits you. If you carry your diary in your handbag you can make notes of what you've eaten wherever you go. You'll also be able to make a note of new recipe ideas or tips as you come across them.

Every day you need to write in your diary what exercise you have done, everything you've had to eat (and we mean everything: no cheating now!) and how you're feeling.

Over time you'll begin to see patterns emerging. It will soon become obvious how your eating, training, moods and energy levels correlate. This will be motivation in itself and is an extremely powerful tool. You'll be able to see for yourself in black and white how eating the right foods and exercising regularly will make you feel good, not just in the long term, but day to day too. It will empower you to take ownership of your life and flag up the habits you need to change to ensure success.

Try to record in your diary every time you eat, rather than at the end of the day when you may have forgotten something. Don't miss anything out. It might be tempting to 'forget' the odd bag of crisps or 'guesstimate' how much wine you've had, but this defeats the purpose of the diary and won't help you reach your goals. Don't forget: nobody has to see your diary except you unless you want them to.

How Your Diary Might Look

Monday 5 October

Exercise I've done today

What I ate

(Include how much, where you were and who you were with)

How I felt

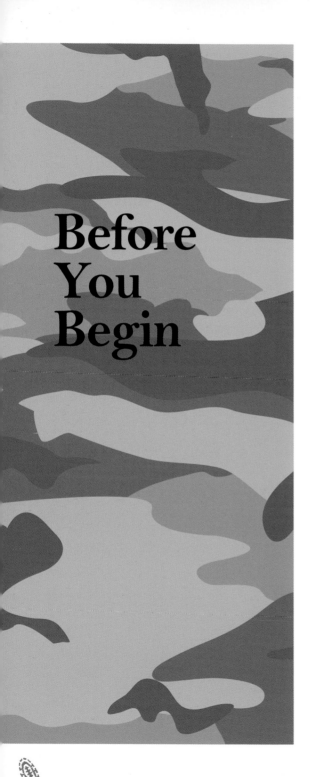

Before You Begin

Sunny and Jacqui's Top Tips for Success

1 Picture your ideal weight. Did you know that there are websites out there that show you exactly how you'll look 10-20-40 or 50lbs lighter? These are great for helping out with your visualizations as they'll give you a very specific picture to focus on. If you can see it, you can achieve it! Try www.weightview.com (it's free). Make sure you print a few copies of your WeightView photo and stick it on your fridge, your mirror and inside your wardrobe.

2 Create a vision board. Think of all the fantastic things you can begin to do as you grow fitter, stronger and more confident. Maybe you're dying to do a triathlon or just want to feel good in your swimsuit on a beach. Cut out a photo of someone winning a race, or relaxing in a fab bikini on an idyllic beach and paste your headshot on top on the photo (come on, don't be shy!). It will help you to believe that it IS possible for you to do all these things and anything else if you put your mind to it.

Hopefully by now you're all fired up and raring to go. Before we pitch in to the two-week Drop-a-Dress-Size plan, we'd like to share a few last tips to help you keep on track. Act on them today to make a flying start to your weight-loss efforts and revisit them whenever you need a boost.

3 Add words to those photos. Maybe put a date under that photo of someone winning a race with a caption that could go along these lines: 'I win my first 10km (6-mile) run by November 15, 20XX!' Remember, the more emotion you put into this, the stronger the connection you will create with your goals.

4 Be flexible. If some part of the programme isn't working for you, then work out why and adapt it.

5 Remember, there is no such thing as failure – only feedback. If you have a bad day, a bad week or even a bad year, don't give up and go back to your old ways. Take note of what you have learned and get back on track to the New You. Although it may not seem like it at the time, failure is possibly one of the best things that can happen to you as it allows you to learn. Everyone fails at one time or another. Don't let it stop you reaching your goals: use it.

6 Find a Boot Camp buddy. If you have big weight-loss goals, why not tell a friend? You'll be surprised how much support you'll get and you never know ... your friend might want to join you and take part in your weight-loss challenge! You're far more likely to stick to the plan if you've got some company. When you feel accountable to someone for goals that you've set for yourself, you'll do your best not to let yourself or the other person down. A bit of friendly competition can work wonders too.

7 When you're thinking positive thoughts you'll feel good and get results. Imagine a future that is interesting, fruitful, healthy and happy and your brain will help you to correlate your behaviour to your thoughts without you even realizing.

8 Take action TODAY. The only way to get to the finish line is to start. Don't procrastinate. Change your life today and start being the New You.

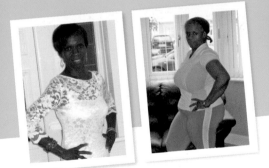

Jacqueline used to weigh 22st 10lbs. She wore a size 32 top and 28–30 bottom. Now Jacqueline weighs around 8st and is a size 8.

Before I lost the weight work was my only comfort. All I did was get up in the morning go to work, work late, do overtime and then go home and eat badly. I hardly went out because I couldn't find nice clothes that fitted and I didn't feel good about myself.

The trigger that convinced me I finally needed to get to grips with my weight was realizing at work one day that I was on my twelfth can of cola and trying to hide the tins. At around the same time I saw a family video of our Christmas dinner. I looked terrible and took up most of the screen. It was so embarrassing. I knew I couldn't carry on like this. First I tried all kinds of fad diets, from pills to shakes and although I lost weight I could never maintain the

loss. I was getting very depressed and didn't know where to turn. Then I heard about gastric banding.

I had a gastric band fitted in 2004 and lost an awful lot of weight but hadn't learned anything about how to eat healthily or exercise. I didn't know what to eat or how to exercise and lacked the confidence to ask for help. I thought that if I went to a gym everyone would be looking at me. I hadn't fundamentally changed the bad habits that had got me into trouble in the first place and I quickly hit a plateau in my weight loss.

Luckily for me I stumbled across a magazine article about Jade Goody and other celebrities attending a weight loss boot camp that promised to kick start weight loss and educate about nutrition and exercise. I knew it was exactly what I needed so I signed up to the New You Boot Camp week. I trained with military trainers and worked with the nutrition squad to devise an exercise and nutrition plan I could use once I had left the camp so all my hard work would not be undone.

'I have lost 14st — over half my body weight!'

I came to New You Boot Camp weighing 12st and wearing a size 16. When I left I weighed 11st 3lbs. New You Boot Camp was the hardest week of my life. If you'd told me before I went that I'd be getting up at 5.30 in the morning and exercising all day until early evening I wouldn't have thought it was possible. Now I know that anything's possible with the right support. Since New You Boot Camp I have continued with the exercise and now know what to eat. I have lost more weight, taking me down to 8st. Sunny and Jacqui are like my family now: they're always there when I'm feeling down or need encouragement. I wish I'd met them before the band was fitted as they provided the education I was lacking!

Everything in my life has changed since I lost the weight. Now I have so much more confidence. All I do is socialize. I do my workouts, I play netball, umpire, meet up with friends, go to events and anything else I can find. I feel young again. I never used to like having my photo taken when I was bigger, but now I love it. I still can't believe my eyes when I see how much weight I've lost. I'm starting my life all over again. I will always, always, remember how I was and how I looked and I'd like to use this opportunity to help other people who are struggling to lose weight like I was. I'm even considering a new career as a fitness coach or counsellor so I can use my experience to benefit others in the same situation.

Now my next task is to try and get my daughter and her father to train with me once in a while, but that is another chapter in my life.

Thank you Sunny and Jacqui for your constant on-going support after New You Boot Camp. Thank you for believing in me and putting me back on track when I went wobbly!

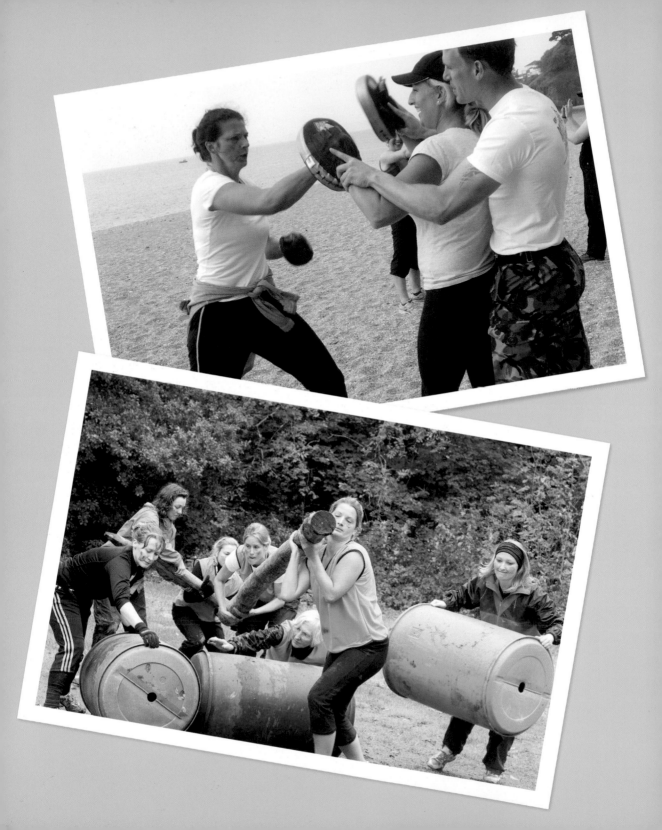

Training

Now you've got your head around what you need to do, it's time to get moving. We're not going to pretend that exercise is ever easy, especially if it's not something that's normally part of your life, but we do believe our programme is manageable for everyone, whether you're a seasoned gym-goer or break out in a sweat at the mere sight of a pair of trainers. You might find it tough at first, but please stick with it. We've seen some incredible transformations at New You Boot Camp, so we know what you can do. As well as helping you to lose weight, finding time to make exercise a habit will give your mood a real boost in the short term and transform your confidence levels.

Why Exercise?

Building regular exercise into your daily routine can be really tough at first, but there's no point fighting it: it has to become a habit. By the end of our Two-Week Drop-a-Dress-Size plan (see page 44), we're confident that you'll be seeing the benefits and may even be starting to enjoy the exercise itself.

Well, maybe not the exercise itself, but at least the rush of feel-good hormones you get straight after a good workout that makes your skin tingle and gives you that burst of self-confidence that leaves you on top of the world. (If you don't know what we mean now, you soon will!)

The good news is that along with earning yourself a fantastic body, if you stick to the New You Boot Camp exercise programme you'll be future-proofing your body and reducing your risk of:

- **HEART DISEASE** Your heart, like any other muscle, gets stronger when trained. This strength allows the heart to pump more blood in every beat, so it has to do less work to get the same result, and is placed under less strain day to day.

- **HIGH CHOLESTEROL** Regular exercise boosts the level of good cholesterol in your blood and lowers the level of bad cholesterol, reducing the risk of strokes and heart attacks and helping to lower your blood pressure.

- **DIABETES** Regular exercise will help control your weight and so reduce your risk of diabetes. It also makes your body more sensitive to insulin and helps to keep your blood sugar levels stable.

- **CANCER** Studies have shown that exercise can reduce the risk of certain cancers by 20–40%.

How Much is Enough?

To stay healthy, the recommended minimum is 30 minutes of light to moderate exercise every day. This can be a walk to work, housework or gardening. You don't have to do 30 minutes all at once, but can split it through the day into three bouts of 10 minutes or even six bouts of 5 minutes.

The bad news is that if you want to shift weight fast that just isn't going to be enough. If you want to burn fat and lose pounds you're going to have to up the intensity. We suggest:

- Duration – About an hour

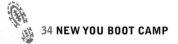

- Frequency – five times per week

- Intensity – 60–85% of Maximum Heart Rate (MHR).

Your Maximum Heart Rate (MHR) is 220 minus your age. So if, for example, you're 40, 220 - 40 = 180. If you want to work at 60% intensity your heartbeats per minute should be no more than 108 when exercising (60 ÷ 100 x 180). Using the same equation, if you want to work at 85% intensity, your heart would beat at no more than 153 beats per minute (85 ÷ 100 x 180). See page 42 for how to measure your pulse when at rest and during a workout.

Top Tips to Get the Most out of Exercise

Drink plenty of water – a dehydrated body functions less efficiently. Aim for at least 2–3 litres (3½–5 pints) a day.

Limit your caffeine to one or two caffeinated drinks a day. This boosts energy and mental alertness. Try fruit teas or redbush tea.

Eat breakfast – food boosts your metabolism and gives the body energy to burn. The brain relies on glucose for fuel, so choose a carbohydrate-rich breakfast (your body breaks carbs down into glucose). Porridge and berries or scrambled egg and salmon on rye toast should do the trick.

Don't overeat or skip meals as both will drain your energy. Spread your food intake more evenly. This will result in more constant blood sugar and insulin levels and so more energy for exercise. You'll also find it easier to lose excess body fat if you eat this way.

Make sure you get enough sleep – the average adult needs about eight hours sleep a night. Make the necessary changes to ensure you get a good night's sleep.

Don't forget to fill out your New You Boot Camp diary with details of all your exercise, so you can see how great it makes you feel.

Make Time to Train

We've worked with enough women to know that by now lots of you are rolling your eyes in disbelief and complaining that we don't understand your busy lives. We know you think you've barely got time to shave your legs, let alone fit in an hour's exercise five times a week. But bear with us.

We're going to ask you to make a leap of faith. Not faith in us, but faith in yourself. We're going to ask you to **make** time. You'll only be able to do this if you believe wholeheartedly that you deserve to be slimmer, fitter and healthier and realize that it's time to stop making excuses and start making time for yourself. At the risk of repeating ourselves, there are no short cuts. So if you want to reach your goals you have no choice but to take a good long look at your schedule and find the time to dedicate to improving your lifestyle.

You will have to be realistic about this. If you're the kind of person who hates getting up in the morning, there's no point in saying you're going to go for a run before work. It just won't happen and you'll feel as though you've let yourself down every day. Equally, if you're always exhausted by the time you get home from work you're unlikely to be able to stick to a plan of exercising in the evening. You might find going for a run round the park at lunchtime fits into your day and lifts you for the afternoon. Fill in the chart opposite and you'll be able to see how your day is spent. But be prepared to make some changes to find the time to make this work. Something's got to give: you just have to decide what it will be.

Don't Give Up!

Exercising regularly isn't easy. There will always be days when you'd rather do anything other than go for a run or do a workout. Research shows that more than 50% of people who begin a fitness programme give up after six weeks. Don't be one of those people. Keep going even when it's hard, and even when you've missed a few days. The following tips should help:

- **SUPPORT** Involve family or friends. It's always better to have a partner to train with.

- **VARY YOUR ROUTINE** Chop and change your exercise routine to maintain the challenge and prevent you from reaching a plateau.

FUN Training doesn't have to mean hours in the gym. Playing a sport, such as tennis or golf, with a friend will introduce some friendly competition and increase the intensity of your workout.

REMEMBER YOUR GOALS Don't lose sight of why you're training. Look back on your Personal Commitment and goals. Use these as motivation when you feel like quitting.

MUSIC Losing yourself in your favourite tracks can take your mind off the training and keep you going for longer. (But please remember to stay alert and aware of your surroundings if you're training outdoors.)

On the days when you really can't fit in that formal exercise session you can still be more active. Every little helps on the road to the New You!

→ Walk to work
→ Take the stairs instead of the elevator
→ Exercise at low/moderate intensity while watching your favourite TV show
→ Perform an exercise like calf raises when standing in a queue
→ Use your lunch break to go for a walk
→ Throw yourself into housework and gardening

DAILY ACTIVITIES	Hours spent by a typical adult	Hours spent by you
Sleeping	8	
Working	8	
Showering/Dressing	1	
Commuting	1	
Seeing friends and family	2	
Doing hobbies	2	
Cooking and eating	1	
Reading / Watching TV / Other	1	
TOTAL	24	

Get the Gear

For those of you who like to shop (and who doesn't?), this could be the section you've been waiting for. It's not going to cost you a fortune to start on our diet and exercise plan, but we do recommend that you invest in a good non-slip exercise mat (so you can follow the workouts safely), a cheap stopwatch and a dynaband (basically a huge elastic band that you use to work your muscles).

What you'll need

Step – you can improvise with the steps in your home or local park
Set of 3kg, 2kg and 1kg dumbbells – if you don't have dumbbells try using two unopened 2-litre bottles of water
Stopwatch
Exercise mat
Dynaband

You could also use

Bicycle
Rowing machine
Treadmill
Cross trainer

What to Wear

As far as what to wear is concerned, you can start out in an old t-shirt and sweat pants and look forward to upgrading to the latest gym wear as a reward for reaching your goals, or hit the shops before you start if looking the part will make you feel more confident. We wouldn't recommend that you spend too much right now, as hopefully you'll soon be shopping for smaller sizes! Treat yourself to one of the popular fitness magazines to check out the latest styles and find stockists. The right shoes and sports bra are a must (see below) but other than that you can improvise the rest of the equipment you need for now and invest as and when you can afford it.

The Basics

Let's start with the basics. Choose a sports bra that's suitable for the activity you're doing. Look for high impact if

> **Remember that exercise is going to be a non-negotiable part of the New You, so it is worth some investment. Putting your money where your mouth is can be another strong motivator.**

you're running or low impact if you're walking or doing yoga. If you intend to do a bit of all three, then cater for the highest-impact sport. Make sure your bra supports you without being too tight. Lots of high street shops offer a bra fitting service and can give you advice if you're not sure what size you need.

- Even more important than your bra are your shoes. We can't stress this enough: if you don't spend money on anything else, then spend money on the right trainers. This applies whatever activity you choose to do, but is particularly important if you're planning on running. The choice is bewildering, so head for a specialist shop who will analyse your gait (the way your weight falls on your feet) for you and steer you towards shoes that will provide the right kind of support and help prevent injuries and joint damage.

- Look for clothes that will be comfortable and practical as you work out. The latest fabrics are designed to manage sweating and temperature control. They draw moisture away from your body to evaporate and keep you warm in winter and cool in summer.

- When exercising it's a good idea to start off wearing several layers so you can peel them off when you're warmed up. You might wear a t-shirt with a hoodie on top that you can take off. If exercising outside, a weatherproof layer on top will protect you from the elements.

- One in four women over the age of 35 suffers from stress incontinence, and if you're overweight, or have had a baby, you're more likely to be affected. If you find you suffer from small leaks of urine when you exercise, you can improve the problem by practising pelvic floor exercises (squeeze and pull in the muscles around your back passage and vagina, hold and release) as often as possible. In the meantime, don't be embarrassed to use protective pads, sold in chemists and supermarkets. Absorbent and secure, they will allow you to exercise with confidence.

Starting Point

Before you start we're going to take some baseline measurements so you can map your progress as you follow the programme.

What you'll need

→ Watch
→ Pen
→ Your New You Boot Camp diary or somewhere else to note down your results
→ Tape measure
→ Scales

Test 1
Weight and BMI

BMI, or body mass index, is a popular measure of how healthy your weight is for your height. It's a useful guideline but remember that you may be above or below the 'normal' measure and still be a healthy weight. If you are fit and muscular, for example, you may fall into the 'overweight' group since muscle is heavier than fat.

BMI = weight in kilograms divided by your height in metres squared

EXAMPLE
If you weigh 10 stone and are 5ft 6in
Convert the measurements to metric: your weight is 63.5kg; your height 1.7m
Square your height: 1.7 x 1.7 = 2.89m
Divide your weight by your height squared = a BMI of 22

WHAT IT MEANS
Below 18.5 **Underweight**
18.5–24.9 **Normal**
25–29.9 **Overweight**
30+ **Obese**

Ideally your BMI should be between 18.5 and 24.9. If it's higher or lower then visit your doctor to make sure you're fit enough to start this programme and rule out any health problems before you start.

Write down your weight and your BMI on page 42 or in your New You Boot Camp diary. Leave space or create a chart so you can check again and see how they change as you progress towards your New You goals.

Test 2
Body Measurements

A better way to find out whether you're losing fat is to take measurements of different parts of your body. This is a more effective way of seeing how much fat you've lost than by checking your weight or BMI, since muscle is heavier than fat and so as you exercise and build muscle you may actually gain weight, even if you are changing shape and becoming leaner and fitter. If you do this test on a regular basis and note the results you'll be amazed how quickly your body shape starts to change. The measurements to take are chest, waist, hips, thigh and upper arm.

Obviously you want to see all those measurements changing, but as far as your health is concerned the most important measurement is your waist-to-hip ratio (how big your waist is compared to your hips). Carrying extra weight around your middle is particularly dangerous for your health, putting you at increased risk of heart disease and diabetes. To work out

HOW TO MEASURE

CHEST
Place the tape measure around your chest so it runs across your nipples.
WAIST
Place the measure around the waist so it runs around your narrowest point.
HIPS
Measure around the widest point.
THIGH
Measure around the top of the leg where it meets your groin.
UPPER ARM
Measure around the top of your arm so the tape measure is touching the top of your armpit.

your waist-to-hip ratio, measure your waist at its narrowest point. Now measure your hips at their widest point (don't pull the tape measure too tight!). Divide your waist measurement by your hip measurement.

For example, if your waist measures 74cm and your hips 95cm:

$$74 \div 95 = 0.78$$

So your ratio is 0.78.

If you're a woman and the figure you get is bigger than 0.85 your weight is putting your health at risk; if you're a man you need to aim to keep the figure below 0.9.

Test 3
Resting Heart Rate

The third and last measurement that we're going to take before we get going is your resting heart rate. Measuring your resting heart rate gives you a good indication of your cardiovascular fitness. If your heart is strong it pumps more blood in each beat so needs to beat fewer times a minute to send blood around your body. Do the test first thing in the morning before exercise or stress affects your beats per minute (bpm). Take your pulse at your wrist for 15 seconds using your finger. Multiply the number of heartbeats by four to find beats per minute. A healthy resting heart rate is between 60 and 75 beats per minute.

Write your resting heart rate in your diary with room to add some more measurements later, or on the table on page 43. After a few weeks of exercising your resting heart rate should fall by one or two beats per minute.

DON'T BEGIN THE BOOT CAMP EXERCISES IF

→ You are, or may be, pregnant. Check with your doctor before exercising.
→ You're recovering from an injury.
→ You have a cold or fever or other temporary illness. Rest until you've recovered.

If you need to test your pulse during a workout to find out how hard you're working (see page 52) take a measure over 6 seconds and multiply by 10. As the pulse rate can fluctuate quickly when you're working hard, it's best to measure it over a short time like this before it starts to slow and affects the reading.

Record Your Results

Body Weight

Now	2 Weeks	1 Month	2 Months	3 Months	4 Months	5 Months	6 Months

BMI

Now	2 Weeks	1 Month	2 Months	3 Months	4 Months	5 Months	6 Months

Body Measurements

	Now	2 Weeks	1 Month	2 Months
Chest				
Waist				
Hips				
Thighs				
Upper Arms				

Body Measurements

	3 Months	4 Months	5 Months	6 Months
Chest				
Waist				
Hips				
Thighs				
Upper Arms				

Resting Heart Rate

Now	2 Weeks	1 Month	2 Months	3 Months	4 Months	5 Months	6 Months

The Two-Week Drop-a-Dress-Size Plan

This is where the hard work really starts! We've designed a programme of cardio (pulse raising) and strength (muscle building) workouts that you can combine to be as rigid or as flexible as you want. To get the best results from the plan you should exercise five times a week, and you can either follow the plan we provide or combine any of the three cardio workouts with any of the three strength workouts. It's up to you. Don't worry if you've never exercised before. We'll show you step-by-step how to work safely and effectively.

To get the best results, try to do a mix of all three cardio workouts every week (not the same one over and over again) followed immediately by one of the home workouts when possible. If you don't have time to do both the cardio and the workout at the same time, you can still reach your goals by completing a cardio session in the morning and one of the home workouts in the evening. If you've really only got time to do one, then do one: don't use it as an excuse to do nothing! Don't forget to add a warm up (see page 46–49) and cool down to each workout you do. You must take a break at least one day a week, as your body needs this time to recover. You can follow the plan on the opposite page rigidly, or mix and match the workouts to suit yourself. Just remember, the more effort you put in, the more you'll get back.

Our Two-Week Exercise Plan

WEEK 1	EXERCISE	WEEK 2	EXERCISE
Monday	Cardio 1 + Workout 2	Monday	Cardio 2 + Workout 3
Tuesday	Cardio 3 + Workout 1	Tuesday	Cardio 1 + Workout 1
Wednesday	Cardio 2 + Workout 3	Wednesday	Cardio 2 + Workout 1
Thursday	Cardio 3 + Workout 1	Thursday	Cardio 3 + Workout 2
Friday	REST	Friday	REST
Saturday	Cardio 1 + Workout 2	Saturday	Cardio 1 + Workout 3
Sunday	REST/Long walk	Sunday	REST/Long walk

For each workout there are three different levels of exercises. If you're a beginner and haven't done much exercise before, go for the Beginners workout. If you're finding that too easy, move on to Intermediate, and if you're already very fit and want to try the more challenging versions of the exercises, go straight to the Tough

Alternative. Each workout focuses on a particular area of the body so we recommend you vary your exercise to get a balanced workout.

To learn how to do our fat-busting cardio workouts go to pages 50-53 and for the strength workouts go to pages 54-79.

Warm Ups

Your warm up is a vital part of your workout. Never be tempted to skip it as it prepares your body physically and mentally for the session ahead. Once you get into the workouts you're going to be working really hard, but if you do your warm up right you'll find the transition from gentle effort to hard exercise much easier than jumping straight into your workout.

What Does the Warm Up Do?

- Increases blood flow to the muscles
- Improves flexibility
- Improves muscle contraction
- Brings better flow of synovial fluid within the joints, which helps movement
- Can help to prevent muscle and joint injury

General Warm Up

We're going to start with gentle movements of the entire body. This raises your heart rate, increases body temperature and mobilizes the main joints that you're going to use during your workout. Break your general warm up down into these stages:

- First pulse raiser
- Stretch and mobilize
- Second pulse raiser

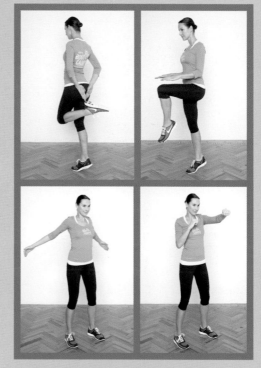

First Pulse Raiser

Start with 2 minutes of gentle jogging, heel flicks, small knee raises, arm circles and arm flicks, as well as side-stepping and light skipping.

Stretch and Mobilize

A good stretch will loosen up your muscles and prepare them for vigorous exercise. Repeat each of the stretches given here twice and hold each one for no more than 10 seconds.

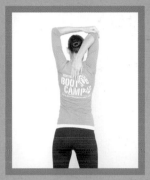

Tricep Stretch

Stand upright with your feet shoulder-width apart. Raise one arm above your head and place the palm of that hand onto the area between your neck and shoulder blades with the elbow pointing towards the ceiling. Bring the other arm up and cup your elbow with your hand. Gently push the elbow backwards to stretch. Repeat on the other side.

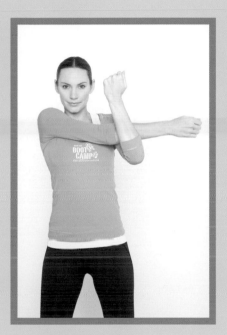

Shoulder Stretch

Stand upright with your feet slightly wider than shoulder-width apart. Extend your right arm straight across your chest. Bring the other arm up and gently ease your right arm in towards your chest. To increase the stretch, turn your head to look over your right shoulder. Repeat on the other side.

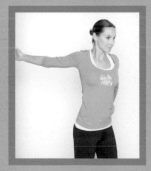

Chest Stretch

Standing in front of a door frame with your left leg forwards and your left hand on your hip, reach back with your right hand and grip the frame. Lean forwards to stretch the chest. Repeat to the other side.

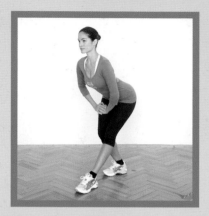

Hamstring Stretch

Bend one knee and extend the other leg out in front. Both sets of toes should be pointing forwards. Bend at your hips and place both hands onto the bent knee. To increase the stretch, raise the toes up. Repeat on the other side.

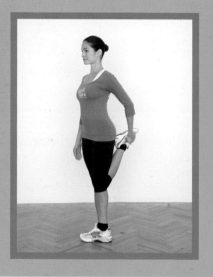

Quadriceps Stretch

Stand upright with your feet together. Lift one foot backwards towards your backside and grasp the front of your foot with the hand on the same side. Bend the other leg slightly at the knee and push your hips forwards, keeping your knees together. Repeat on the other side. (If you have trouble balancing, you can lean against a wall with your free hand to support yourself while you're doing this stretch.)

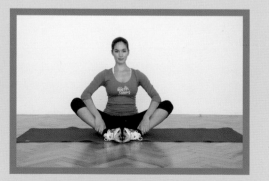

Adductor Stretch

Sit down and bring the soles of your feet together, allowing your knees to fall outwards so your legs make a diamond shape. Place your elbows into the insides of your knees and push the legs downwards to stretch the adductors.

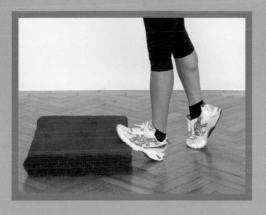

Calf Stretch

Place your toes onto a low step and drop your heel down towards the ground. Repeat on the other side.

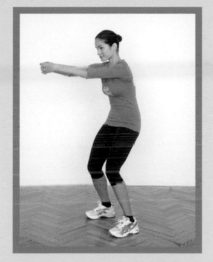

Upper Back Stretch

Stand upright with your feet shoulder-width apart. Extend both arms out in front of you at shoulder height. Clasp your hands together and tuck your chin in towards your chest. Push forwards with your hands.

Second Pulse Raiser

Now do the same as you did for your first pulse raiser, but really put some welly into it this time. You're aiming to get out of breath now. You can also add activities like sprinting on the spot and jumping. Do this for another 2 minutes.

Specific Warm Up

If you have time, you can add a specific warm up, which should include things you're going to do during your main workout. For example, if you are about to run you should do a pulse raiser as above and then jog lightly on the spot for a few minutes, or you could do a couple of reps of the exercises in your workout.

The Cardio Workouts

A cardiovascular workout is one that gets your heart working. It can take lots of different forms, but always involves using the body's largest muscle groups in a repetitive way over a period of time to raise your heart rate.

Top Tip

Whatever sport you choose for your cardio workout, pay attention to your posture. Try to keep your shoulders relaxed and your stomach lightly drawn in to support your back muscles and prevent injury. If you're running, don't clench your hands into fists as this creates tension throughout your body.

You can do things that you're already familiar with such as aerobics, skipping, walking, jogging and cycling. If you regularly go to the gym you can perform your cardio workouts on the treadmill or cross trainer. When you need to break out of your comfort zone try new activities such as boxing or playing netball — there are so many possibilities. In our two-week plan we've included three different ways to carry out your cardio workout, as varying the way you work is the best way to improve your fitness levels and avoid hitting plateaus where you don't feel you're making any progress.

Steady State

Steady state exercise is performed at a steady, even pace that is at a low enough level to allow you to maintain the same speed for prolonged periods. At this pace you should be able to hold a conversation without getting out of breath.

Interval Training

When you're interval training you perform your activity (running, rowing, cycling, etc.) at near maximum effort with periods of rest or low activity to let you recover in between efforts. The recovery period is often short, and this is a great way to build up your fitness levels.

Fartlek Training

Although it sounds a bit dodgy, Fartlek is actually Swedish for 'speed play' and simply means that you vary your pace throughout your workout. If you're running, for example, you might set out at a steady lick, sprint as hard as you can for a couple of minutes, then slow to a jog until you've got your breath back, before going through the whole process again. This sort of training is very flexible, as you can work at your own individual pace, and can be really good fun. If you feel nervous about really going for it and working hard, this is a good option to choose since you can try it out in short bursts and recover at your own pace.

CARDIO 1
Steady State

For your first cardio workout you need to do 30–50 minutes of exercise. It can be any form of exercise that raises your heart rate, so you could start with an outdoor run, or if you like going to the gym this could be a run on the treadmill or a stint on the cross trainer. Try mixing it with cycling or swimming. Keep things interesting by trying out other activities like hill walking, rock climbing, horseriding or canoeing. This should be performed at 65% of MHR or at level 5 on the RPE scale. Remember, this means that although you're working moderately hard you should still be able to hold a conversation. Don't go hell for leather for the first five minutes then find you can't keep up your pace. If you haven't exercised before then take things slowly to start with and as you get fitter you can pick up your pace.

CARDIO 2
Interval Training

You can use this programme for whatever activity you prefer: running, cycling, cross-training, a session on a rowing machine, or anything else that gets your heart pumping. Don't forget, you need to be working flat out, as hard as you possibly can, over the distances given, then rest for the time stated before starting off again. This should take between 30 and 50 minutes. It's a tough workout so you'll need lots of grit and determination to see it through. Don't forget, the more you do it the easier it gets. Remind yourself of your New You Boot Camp goals and go for it.

RPE (rate of perceived exertion) LEVEL	DISTANCE	REST PERIOD
Exercise for 5 minutes at RPE level 4		
10	100 metres	30 seconds
10	200 metres	60 seconds
10	300 metres	90 seconds
10	400 metres	120 seconds
10	500 metres	150 seconds
10	400 metres	120 seconds
10	300 metres	90 seconds
10	200 metres	60 seconds
10	100 metres	FINISH
Exercise for 5 minutes at RPE level 4		

CARDIO 3
Fartlek Training

Complete 40 minutes of exercise. As with the steady state cardio workout, this can be done using any form of exercise that raises your heart rate. We've given you an example of how to vary your effort here, but once you get the hang of it you can play with it to suit yourself. This is a very informal type of workout and one that you can have a lot of fun with once you've built up your confidence.

TIME	EFFORT
1 minute	50% of Max effort or RPE Level 5
1 minute	60% of Max effort or RPE Level 6
30 seconds	80% of Max effort or RPE Level 8
Continue for 40 minutes (repeating the cycle 16 times)	

The Strength Workouts

Now we come to our New You Boot Camp strength workouts. Just to remind you why it's such a good idea to combine strength-building exercises with your cardio workout, these exercises will tone your body, giving you your best shape ever and by building muscle will increase the rate at which you burn fat, even when you're asleep. Each workout focuses on a different part of the body, so for a balanced result we'd recommend that you do all three. If you have a particular problem area that you'd like to address you can repeat the relevant workout a few extra times. Turn to pages 56–65 to see detailed step-by-step instructions for how to perform each exercise.

You might find that your muscles get tired and ache while you're completing the workouts; that's perfectly normal and will improve as your fitness levels increase, but if you feel any sharp pains then **STOP** straight away and rest. Check that you're performing the exercise correctly before you try again.

Workout 1 – Upper Body

Perform each exercise the number of times stated in the chart. Once you've done each exercise the given number of times, rest for 1 minute and repeat the whole process for the second set. Rest for 1 minute and then complete the final set.

	BEGINNERS	INTERMEDIATE	ADVANCED (Tougher Alternatives)
Press Ups	10	12	10
Lateral Raise	12	14	10
Tricep Dips	12	16	14
Bicep Curls	12	16	14
Shoulder Press	12	14	12
Bent Over Row	10	12	10
Sets	3	3	3

Workout 2 – Abs and Back

Perform each exercise the number of times stated in the chart. Once you've done each exercise the given number of times, rest for 1 minute and repeat the whole process for the second set. Rest for 1 minute and then complete the final set.

	BEGINNERS	INTERMEDIATE	ADVANCED (Tougher Alternatives)
Bridge	10	12	12
Half Sit	16	20	16
Dorsal Raise	10	12	12
Plank	20 seconds	30 seconds	30 seconds
V-Sits	16	20	16
Superwoman	10 each side	12 each side	12 each side
Sets	3	3	3

Workout 3 – Lower Body

Perform each exercise the number of times stated in the chart. Once you've done each exercise the given number of times, rest for 1 minute and repeat the whole process for the second set. Rest for 1 minute and then complete the final set.

	BEGINNERS	INTERMEDIATE	ADVANCED
Deadlifts	12	14	14
Lunges	10 each leg	12 each leg	12 each leg
Side Lying Leg Raise	12 each leg	14 each leg	14 each leg
Squats	14	18	16
Calf Raise	20	25	25
Sumo Squat	12	16	16
Sets	3	3	3

Strength Exercises

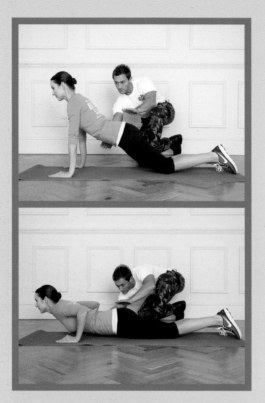

For maximum effectiveness you should work with the heaviest weights you can safely manage. Where we have recommended a 2 or 3kg weight and you find this tough, you can start with a lower weight and increase it as soon as you are able to manage it. Always work within your capabilities to avoid injury.

Press Up on Knees

Start in a full press up position and lower your knees to the floor. Keeping your back straight, bend your arms and lower your chest towards the floor. Straighten your arms without locking them out.

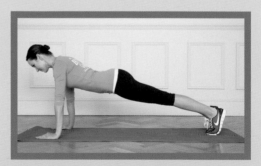

Tough Alternative

Perform full press ups with straight legs and toes tucked under.

Lateral Raise

Stand with your feet shoulder-width apart and hold a 2kg dumbbell (or 2-litre water bottle) in each hand. Maintain a slight bend in your arms and extend your arms out to the sides until they are slightly higher than shoulder height. Now lower your arms down until the weights are by your side and then repeat.

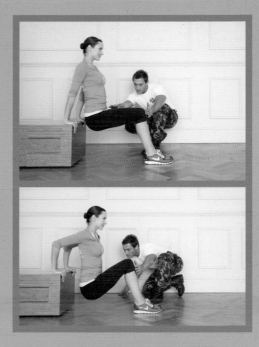

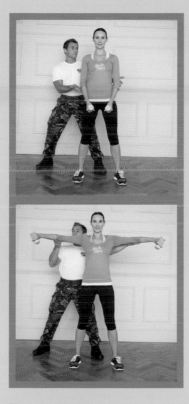

Tough Alternative

Hold arms out at shoulder height for 3 seconds between each repetition.

Tricep Dips

Sit on the edge of a step box or heavy chair and hold on to the edge. Move your bottom off the edge of the box or chair, keeping your feet flat on the floor. Your backside should be level with the box. Gently lower your backside towards the floor so your arms take the strain. Lower until your elbows are at a 90-degree angle and then raise back up to the starting position.

Tough Alternative

Perform tricep dips with straight legs.

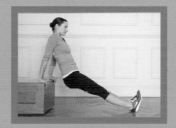

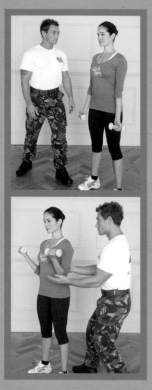

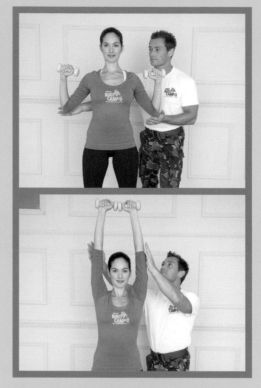

Bicep Curl

Stand with your feet shoulder-width apart with a slight bend in your knees. Hold a dumbbell (or 2-litre water bottle) in each hand and keep your arms close by your side. Keep your elbows locked in to the side of the body and bend your forearm, bringing the dumbbell up to shoulder height. Lower and repeat.

Tough Alternative

Once at the top of the repetition, take 4 seconds to lower the dumbbells back to the starting position.

Shoulder Press

Standing with feet shoulder-width apart, hold a dumbbell in each hand at shoulder height, palm facing forwards. Extend your arms upwards, keeping the dumbbells close together.

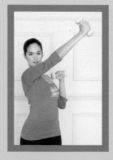

Tough Alternative

From the same start position extend one arm diagonally upwards across your chest. Repeat with alternate arms.

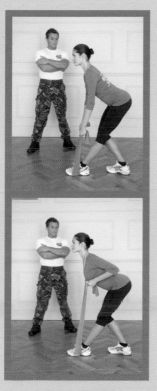

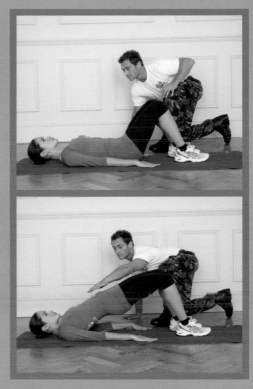

Bent Over Row

Stand with one foot in front of the other and place a dynaband underneath your front foot. Bend over to grasp the ends of the band, bending your back leg and keeping the front leg straight. Pull the ends of the band up towards your chest, keeping your elbows in.

Bridge

Lie on your back with your knees bent to 90 degrees and your feet flat on the floor. Keep your arms by your sides, palms facing down. Gently raise your hips in the air and squeeze your bottom. Hold at the top, then gently lower, ensuring your backside does not touch the floor between repetitions.

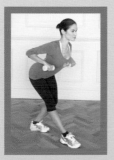

Tough Alternative

Maintaining the same position, perform the exercise with dumbbells instead of a dynaband.

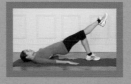

Tough Alternative

Hold at the top and gently straighten one leg at the knee, lower and repeat for the opposite leg.

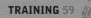

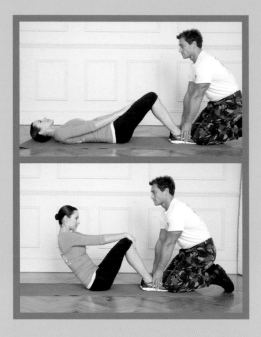

Half Sit

Lie on your back with your knees bent to 90 degrees and your feet flat on the floor. Lay your palms on your thighs, then raise your upper body up until your knee is cupped by the palm of your hand. Gently lower your body down again.

Tough Alternative

Once at the top of the repetition, raise both arms to a vertical position above your head. Lower your arms to your knees and lower your upper body to the ground.

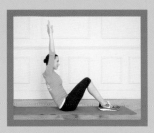

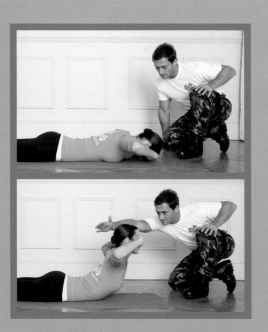

Dorsal Raise

Lie face down, legs together, with your fingertips on your temples. Raise your head and shoulders off the floor and then return to starting position.

Tough Alternative

As you raise up, straighten your arms out in front of you, then bring them out to the sides into the crucifix position before returning your fingertips to your temples.

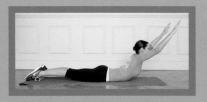

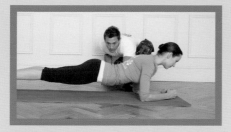

Plank

Lying on your stomach, place the weight of your body onto your forearms and raise your body off the floor with the weight on your toes and forearms. Keep your body parallel to the floor and hold the position for the desired time.

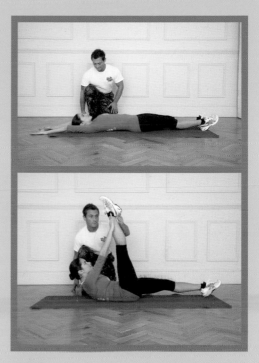

V-Sits

Lie on the floor with your arms and legs extended. Keeping your arms and legs as straight as possible, raise one leg and both arms off the floor and aim to touch your toes with your hands. Gently lower and repeat on the other side.

Tough Alternative

Perform V-sits as above but raise both legs for each repetition.

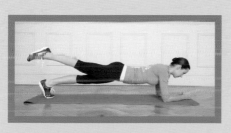

Tough Alternative

Perform the plank as above but raise one leg off the ground. Repeat with the other leg.

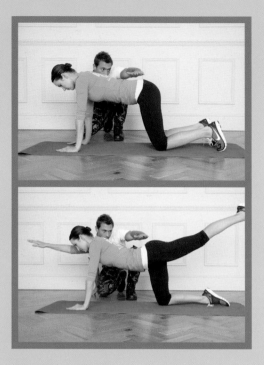

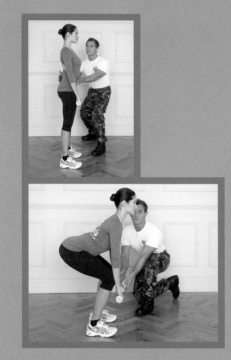

Superwoman

Go on to your hands and knees and gently extend one leg and the opposite arm out until they are parallel with the floor. Slowly bring the arm and leg back and repeat on the other side.

Tough Alternative

Perform Superwoman as above while lying on your stomach.

Deadlifts

Stand upright with a 2kg dumbbell (or 2-litre bottle of water) in each hand and your feet slightly wider than shoulder-width apart. Bend your body forwards and bend your knees, keeping your back straight, and lower the dumbells towards the floor. Then raise back up.

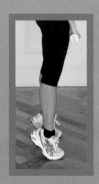

Tough Alternative

Between repetitions, keeping the dumbbells close to your body, raise yourself up onto your toes.

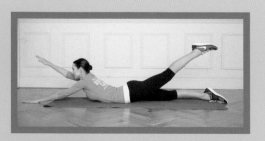

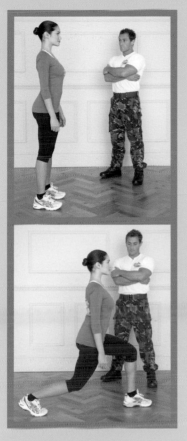

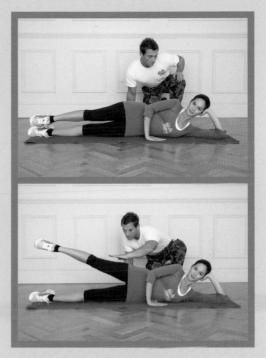

Lunges

Stand upright with your feet together and your arms by your sides. Keeping your back straight, step one leg forwards into the lunge position. Drive the front foot forward, keeping the heel down. The knee behind should almost be touching the floor. Push up to return to the starting position and repeat for the opposite leg.

Tough Alternative

Perform the lunge with a light dumbbell in each hand.

Side Lying Leg Raise

Lie on your side with your legs together with your ankles, knees, hips and shoulders all in one straight line and your head supported by your hand. Gently raise the top leg. Lower and ensure you maintain a 15cm (6in) gap between your feet before the next repetition. Repeat on the other side.

Tough Alternative

Hold each repetition at the top for 3 seconds.

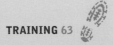

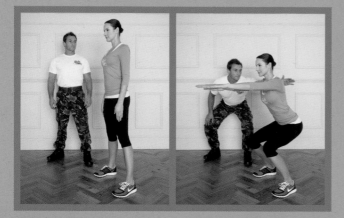

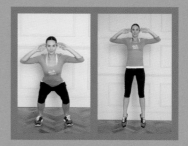

Squats

Stand upright, with your feet slightly wider than shoulder-width apart. With your back straight and your arms out in front and parallel with the ground, push your backside out as though you were about to sit on a chair. Lower yourself into a squat, keeping your head up and chest out, then push up with your legs to come back up to standing.

Tough Alternative

Add a jump in between each repetition.

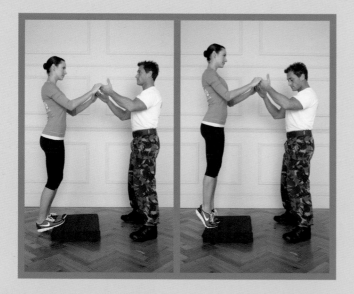

Calf Raise

Stand with your heels on the floor and your toes raised on an object (such as a book). Slowly raise your heels off the ground and put the weight onto the balls of your feet. Lower gently back down.

Tough Alternative

Count to 4 seconds before gently lowering your heels to the ground.

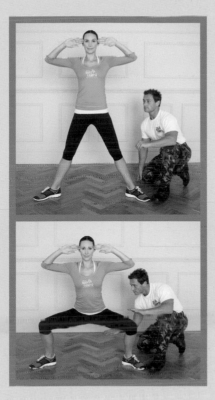

Sumo Squats

Stand with your feet approximately 1m (1yd) apart with your toes facing outwards and your hands by your temples. Lower down into the squat position.

Tough Alternative

Perform the adductor squats as above but with a dumbbell held in front of you in each hand.

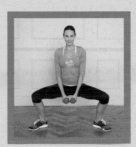

COOL DOWN

Well done! You've got to the end of a tough workout. You might feel like collapsing in a heap on the floor, but first you really need to cool down. This will give your body the chance to return gradually to a steady state and shift any build up of lactic acid and waste products that are still in your bloodstream from exercising. If you don't cool down properly you're more likely to feel sore for a couple of days after exercising. This is known as Delayed Onset of Muscle

Soreness or DOMS. It's perfectly normal and should disappear within 48 hours. It's definitely NOT an excuse to duck out of your next training session.

To cool down, simply repeat the first pulse raiser of the warm up. Then run through the stretches (go back to pages 46–49 to see how to stretch), holding each one for no more than 10 seconds. To get the best results, make your cool-down last for about 5–10 minutes.

What Next?

Wow! You made it! You've completed the Two-Week Drop-a-Dress-Size plan. Give yourself a huge cheer and find a treat to reward your efforts (but not one you can eat).

The At Home Circuits

We're sure you've already reached for the tape measure and the scales and can see the pounds and inches dropping off: don't forget to record your achievements. If you've stuck faithfully to the plan you'll have seen some impressive results. If you found it tough going and wobbled more than you'd like to admit, then don't despair. Any efforts you have made will have made a difference, even if that's not as obvious as you'd like. You've started on the road to the New You and there's no turning back now. The Boot Camp at Home circuits that follow are designed to be used on an ongoing basis, 3–4 times per week to keep you fit and trim for life. You can mix and match them as you like, and even continue to use the workouts you're used to if you want some variety. You should try to keep up the cardio workouts as well and eat according to our Four-Step Plan (see pages 84–85). Keep looking back at your Personal Commitment and the goals you've set to remind yourself why you're making the effort.

Circuit 1
The Stair

What to do

This is an aerobic circuit.
Do 10 repetitions of each exercise.
Between each exercise run up, down, then up the stairs (or down, up, then down).
So you start with the first exercise at the bottom of the stairs, the next exercise will be at the top, the third at the bottom and so on.

Rest for one minute between circuits and repeat twice more.

What You'll Need

1 x dynaband

1 x set of 3kg dumbbells (use two 2-litre water bottles if you don't have dumbbells)

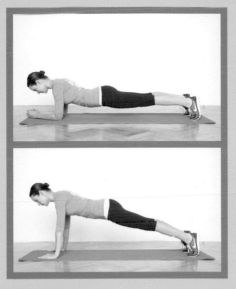

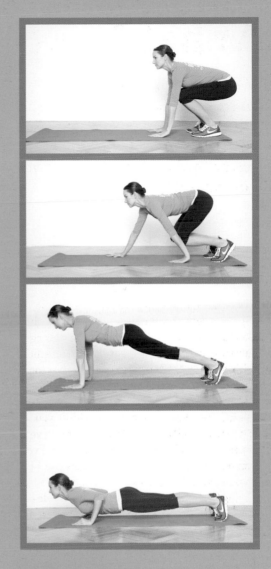

Plank/Press

Lying on your stomach, place the weight of your body onto your forearms and raise your body off the floor with the weight on your toes and forearms. From there push up from your forearms, step your hands back and place your palms on the floor so you are in the full press-up position. Lower from the press-up position back into the plank. Repeat 10 times.

Walkaways

Stand upright, feet together. Bend your knees, place your hands on the floor, walk your body out until you are in the press-up position. Perform a press-up and walk back to the upright position. Repeat 10 times.

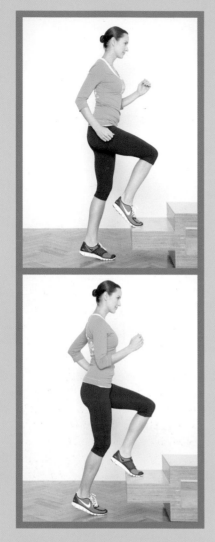

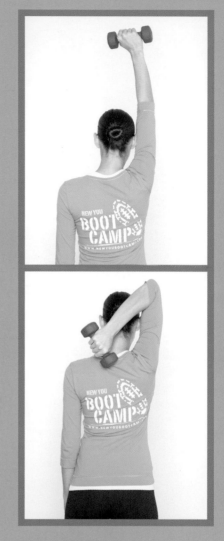

Toe Tapping

Stand in front of the bottom step of the stairs. Jump and tap alternate toes onto the bottom step. Try to get a rhythm going. Repeat 10 times.

Tricep Press

Stand with your back straight and a slight bend in your knees. Hold a dumbbell in one hand and raise it straight above your head. Keeping your elbow still, bend and lower the weight behind your head then gently raise it back up. Complete 10 repetitions on each arm.

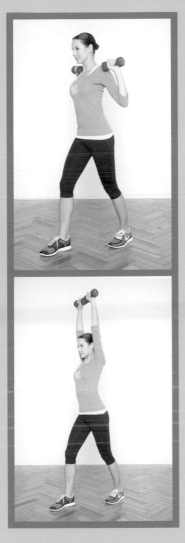

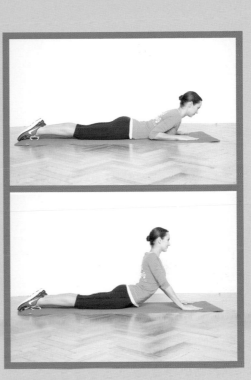

Dorsal Press

Lie on your stomach, legs together and hands by your shoulders. Push up from your arms until your arms are straight and then gently lower yourself back to the floor. Repeat 10 times.

Shoulder Press

Standing upright, place one foot in front of the other. Hold a dumbbell in each hand at shoulder height. Raise them both above your head, gently tap the dumbbells together and lower. Repeat 10 times.

 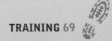

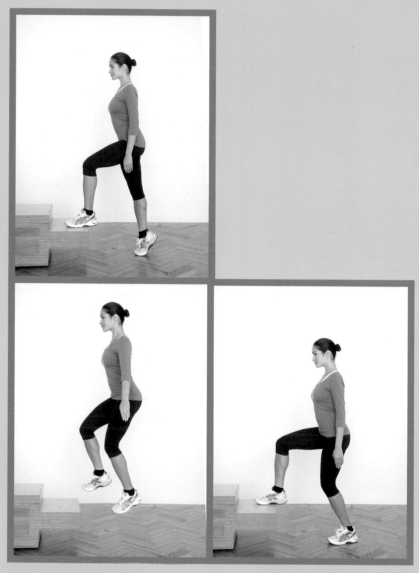

Stair Split Jumps

Start with one foot on the bottom step of the stairs. Use that leg to push up and jump into the air. While you are in the air, change legs so the other leg lands on the bottom step. Repeat 10 times for each leg.

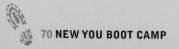

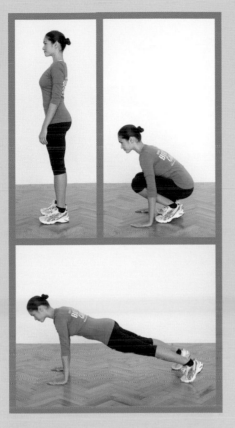

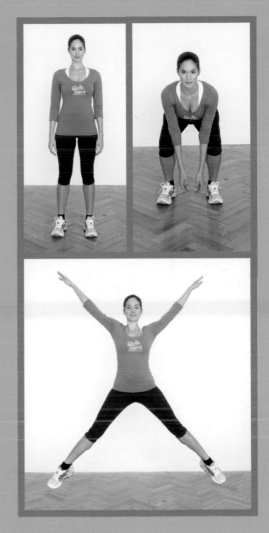

Burpees

Stand upright, feet together. Bend down, place both hands on the floor and jump both legs out behind you so you are in the press-up position. Now jump both knees back into the chest and stand upright. Repeat 10 times.

Star Jumps

Stand upright with feet together. Bend down into the crouch position and then jump up with arms and legs outstretched. Bring your arms and legs back into the midline as you lower back down into the crouch position ready for the next repetition. Repeat 10 times.

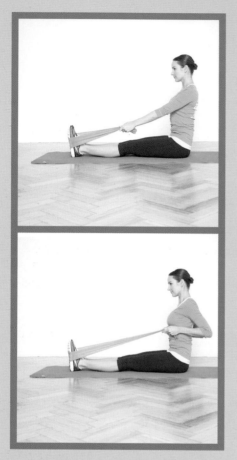

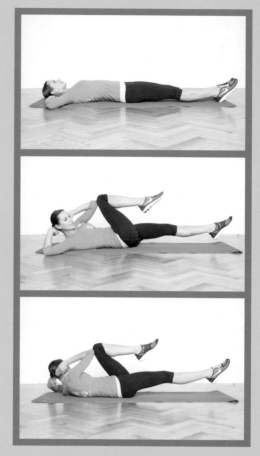

Seated Row

Sit down, with your legs straight out in front of you and your back upright. Place the dynaband around the soles of your feet. Open your legs to place tension on the band. Keeping the handles close to your body, pull your elbows in and past your torso, attempting to squeeze your shoulder blades together. Repeat 10 times.

Bicycles

Lie on your back and place your fingertips on your temples or behind your neck. Lift both legs off the floor slightly and bring the one knee in towards your chest. Rotate the elbow on the opposite side to meet the bent knee. Come slowly back to the starting position and repeat for opposite side. Complete 20 in total.

Circuit 2
The Dose

What to do

To complete the Dose Circuit, first you need to work out your own individual 'dose'. You can use the chart below, or copy it into your New You Boot Camp diary. Take 1 minute to complete the maximum number of quality repetitions that you can for each exercise. Correct technique is more important than speed. Rest for 1 minute between exercises. Make a note of the number of repetitions in the number column. Split this number in half and write the score into the dose column. If you score an odd number, then round up to the next even number to work out your dose. Do this once a month to get your dose score.

Once you've recorded a score for each exercise you're ready to get started on the circuit. Work your way through all the exercises, completing the number of repetitions in the dose column. Once you have completed all the exercises, rest for 2 minutes then go through them all again. Complete the whole circuit three times in total.

Record your time for each circuit and remember to re-test and adjust your dose scores every month.

EXERCISE	NO.	DOSE
In, Out, Up, Downs		
Crunch		
Stand Up – Lie Downs		
B52s		
Upright Rows		
Ankle Taps		
Astride Jumps		
Arm Punches		
Reverse Crunch		
Squat Thrusts		
Bum Jumps		

DATE	CIRCUIT TIME

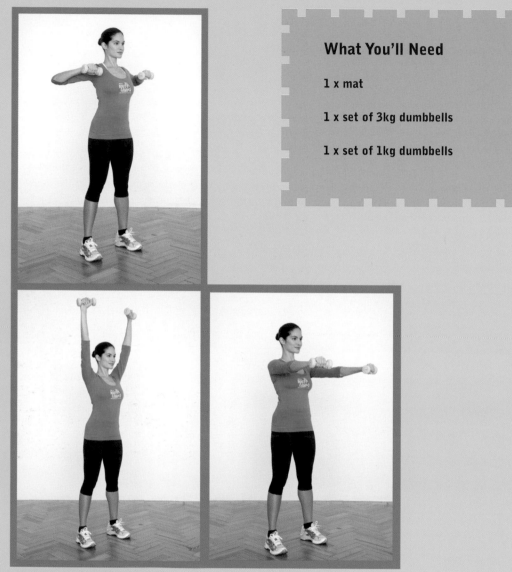

In, Out, Up, Downs

Stand upright with feet shoulder-width apart. Hold a 3kg dumbbell in both hands against your chest. Push the dumbbell away from your body, keeping your arms straight. Take it back in towards your chest, push towards the ceiling and then lower back to its starting position.

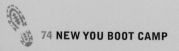

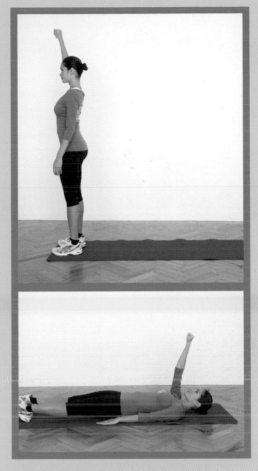

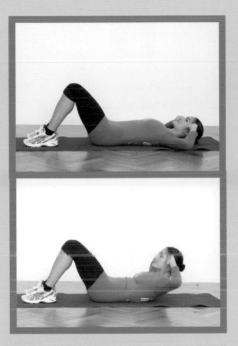

Crunch

Lie on your back with your knees bent to an angle of 90 degrees and your feet flat on the floor. Put your fingers on your temples. Raise your head and shoulders off the floor and then gently lower, allowing only the bottom of your shoulder blades to come into contact with the mat before you raise again.

Turkish Get Up

Lie on your back with one arm by your side and the other raised vertically into the air, hand clenched into a fist. Stand up, keeping your fist pointing vertically upwards at all times. Repeat with the other arm raised.

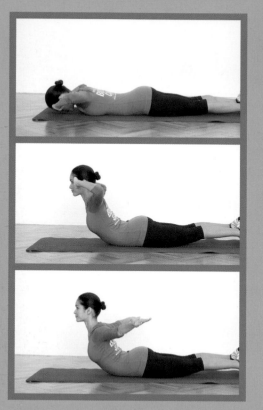

B52s

Lie on your stomach with your fingertips on your temples. Raise your head and shoulders off the mat. Extend your arms to the sides in the crucifix position, then bring your fingertips back to your temples and lower your head and shoulders back to the floor.

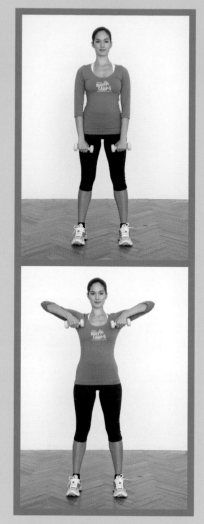

Upright Rows

Stand upright with your feet shoulder-width apart. Hold a dumbbell in each hand in front of your body. Raise the dumbbells up towards your chin and then gently lower.

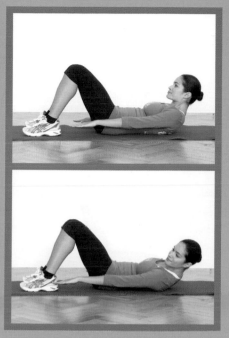

Ankle Taps

Lie on your back with your arms by your side. Lift your head and shoulders off the mat: this is your starting position. Reach down to the side and touch your right ankle with your right hand. Come back to the centre then repeat on the opposite side.

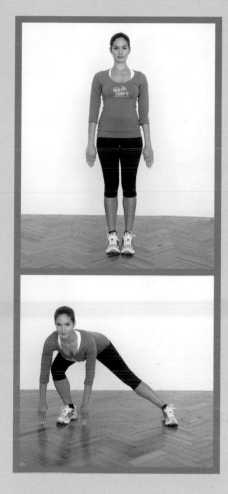

Side Lunge

Stand upright with your feet together and arms by your sides. Take a wide step out to the side with your right foot and bend forwards to touch the floor, keeping your back straight. Return to your start position and repeat to the opposite side.

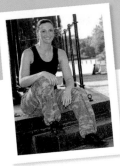

It was while I was reading a magazine that I noticed a story about how Jade Goody had lost weight after going to a boot camp. I needed to lose a bit of weight and fancied doing something similar. There was also a lot going on at work and I needed to get away.... then I spotted an advert for the New You Boot Camp in Wales, and on a whim, I booked it. Our group was picked up from the station by one of the trainers and taken to a farmhouse in the middle of the countryside. After a weigh-in and a fitness test, we were split into groups depending on our fitness levels. The staff ran through a list of rules – such as what time we had to get up (usually 5am) and how two leaders would be instructed to get the rest of the girls downstairs with the correct kit each morning. If we failed, there would be punishments in the form of press-ups, squat thrusts or star jumps.

We'd begin each day by lining up and going for a march before breakfast. From one hour to the next we never knew what we'd be doing, but it ranged from boxing, outdoor circuits, cricket and team sports to walks, team-building exercises such as raft building, and running.

The first three days were the toughest – and we were advised just to focus on getting past these first three day while our bodies adjusted to the regime. We were also given nutritional advice and healthy diets to follow. But I soon got used to it, especially as the two boot camp staff were so good looking! And the group got on brilliantly. On the last day, we did the same fitness test that we'd done at the start of the week, and the results were amazing! Everyone had improved.

Since I've been home, I've had a real spring in my step. I can't bear being inside and I go to the gym four mornings a week before work. It's also boosted my confidence. I feel great – my hair is shiny, my nails are growing and my diet is so much healthier. I've also made some life-long friends and we meet up regularly. New You Boot Camp made me realize that, with a little teamwork, you can do anything – and the brilliant thing is we all want each other to succeed. I've been so inspired that I've even run my first marathon.

Since returning I have lost $9\frac{1}{2}$lbs, $8\frac{1}{2}$ inches and gone from a size 12 to a gorgeous size 8... how good is that! You can't put a price on it! Thank you NYBC team

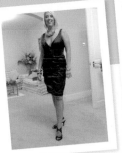
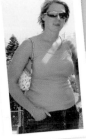

Earlier this year I went on holiday to a hotel I have been to many times. One of the bar staff commented that my body had 'filled out'. We were in the Caribbean and the girls there do say it how it is, but still it hurt! Once at home I went to the doctor as I wasn't sleeping well and felt a bit low. The doctor discovered my blood pressure was high and said it could be due to weight gain amongst other things. He advised me to start doing exercise and have some tests. This was the trigger I needed as I really needed some motivation to get me started. I didn't feel happy about going to a gym in case I saw anyone I knew. Then New You Boot Camp came along. I buy lots of magazines and had read about New You Boot Camp, so I booked myself in. My friends were surprised I was doing it and my parents thought I would be home in a day – I almost was! But I did it and the results have been amazing. I lost 9lbs and 10 inches.

When I got home I joined a gym within 24 hours and have been going almost every day since. I haven't put on any weight, which has given me great confidence, and I can now run 4km on the treadmill! My blood pressure has dropped to a much healthier level and, while I am having tests to find out why it is still a bit high, I feel much less worried about it.

My confidence was tested last week when I was invited as a guest to attend an event that I used to organize in my old job. None of my workmates or clients had seen me since I returned from camp so I put on my new size 10 dress, new heels and off I went. The response was fantastic; I felt great and by the sound of it didn't look so bad either! The fact that my dress was straight and fitted was amazing to my friends, as normally I would go for something that hid my stomach. Not this time...

I will admit New You Boot Camp was the hardest thing I have ever done and if my car had been there I would have gone home on Day Two, but I am so pleased I didn't. It was worth every penny, every tear and every pair of tracksuit bottoms! There is still a way to go with my weight and toning up but I feel so much better. I'm in a position to do the stuff I should have done years ago but didn't have the courage to do then. Now I feel I do... as long as I pack my trainers I think I'll be just fine.

Thank you New You Boot Camp.

It was worth every penny, every tear and every pair of tracksuit bottoms!

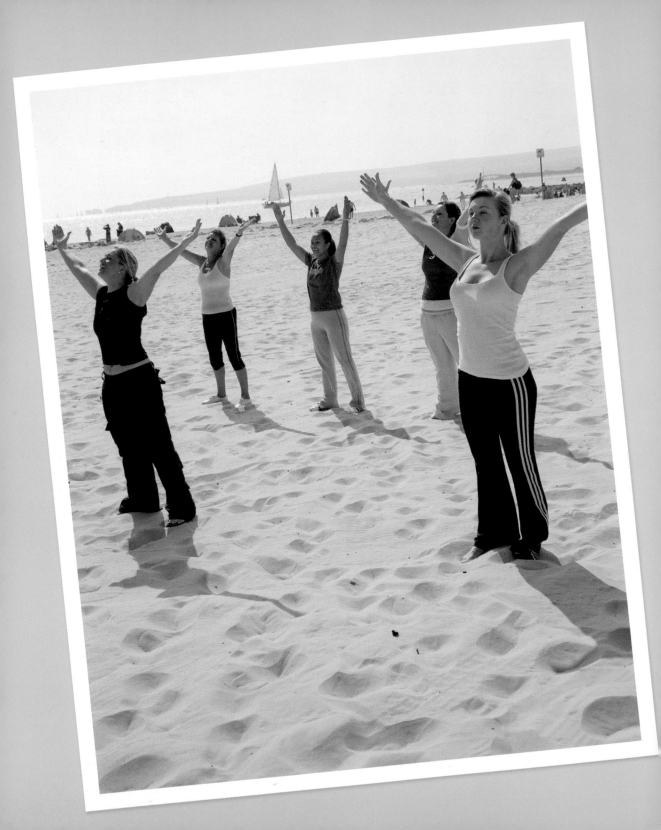

Nutrition

We devised our New You Boot Camp eating plan with two aims in mind: to help you to reach and maintain a healthy weight and to free you from the tyranny of endless dieting. We're not going to call it a diet, and it's essential that you don't think of it as a diet. It's a way of eating that will allow your body to find its own balance, do away with hunger pangs and cravings and help you reach your ideal weight. If you follow our strict two-week eating plan and combine it with exercise you can expect to drop a dress size in that time. The menus are carefully balanced so you won't feel hungry. We've made it easy to make healthy choices, so you'll have plenty of opportunity to celebrate success and feel good about yourself, and once the two weeks are up you can easily adapt the plan to provide a sustainable way of eating that will keep you slim and healthy for life.

The New You Boot Camp Four-Step Plan

The bedrock of the New You Boot Camp programme is our simple four-step eating plan. This will show you how to enjoy your food and nurture your body for life, both while you're losing weight and when you're at your ideal weight.

We've included a two-week wheat- and dairy-free menu that's designed to help you drop between 4–10lbs in two weeks (see pages 100–103). But that's really just our way of holding your hand as you take your first steps along the road to a whole new way of eating. If you prefer, you can skip the menus and go straight to eating whatever you fancy within the New You Boot Camp rules. As long as you combine it with our exercise plan and stay within the rules we promise you'll still enjoy impressive weight loss and unprecedented energy levels. So, let's get on and do it …

Four Steps to Freedom

Step 1   Eat three meals a day and two snacks

No more, but no less either. Forget about trying to deprive yourself or skipping meals. It doesn't work! Don't leave more than three hours between meals/snacks. If you don't eat regularly your metabolic rate goes down: missing out on one meal a day will slow your metabolism down by 15%. You'll lose more weight eating selectively than you will by fasting, so get eating!

Step 2   Choose freely from our Free Foods list

The majority of the foods you eat throughout the day should come from the list of Free Foods on page 88. We don't ask you to weigh your food or count anything, but it is important that you follow our palm-sized portion advice (see page 88).

Step 3
Add Protein Foods, Fabulous Fruit and Healthy Options

You should include some protein from the Protein Foods list at every meal and snack. The body has to work hard to digest protein so it uses up calories and increases your metabolic rate. It also slows the release of sugar into your bloodstream. At every meal you should have one palm-sized portion of protein and at every snack you should have one tablespoon-sized portion. Nuts and seeds are the exception to this: although they're a healthy source of protein and other nutrients, they're high in fat, so you should never eat more than two to three tablespoon-sized portions per day.

In addition to the Free Foods and your Protein Foods, you are allowed to choose up to two portions of fruit and two healthy options from the Healthy Options list on page 90 a day. These are medium- and low-GI carbohydrates (see pages 86–87) that will fill you up without sending your blood sugar levels soaring.

Step 4
After the first two weeks you can choose a cheat day or follow the 80/20 rule

Because we don't expect you to be perfect, after the first two weeks you're allowed to choose to have one cheat day a week or follow the 80/20 rule throughout the week.

If you choose a cheat day you can have one day a week to eat your favourite foods. As

well as helping you not to feel deprived, having a cheat day will remind you how your body feels after you have eaten rubbish. You'll feel sluggish and lethargic, and less inclined to cheat on the plan for the rest of the week. You still need to exercise restraint and stick to three meals and two snacks, and palm-sized portions, but you can include some of the foods that are not allowed on the plan, such as wheat and dairy. Your cheat day is useful if you know you've got a big occasion coming up: a wedding or party when you know there'll be lots of temptation around. Don't sit in a corner feeling deprived. Go for it knowing that you're still following the rules to the letter. But don't forget, if you choose this option, no slacking for the rest of the week!

If you choose to follow the 80/20 rule throughout the week, you stick to the plan 80% of the time and slacken off for 20%. So, out of the 21 meals you have in a week you can include restricted foods such as wheat and dairy in four of them, and perhaps have a glass of wine too. If you've stuck to your plan for the rest of the day you can afford a little indulgence.

Please don't think that you can speed things up by dispensing with this step. Everyone needs a cheat day or 80/20 rule or you'll feel that you're in diet hell. Also, it means that you can have a wobble, or just a treat, without feeing that you've fallen off the wagon and beating yourself up about it. Feeling good is what this plan is about.

Just remember that you CAN'T do both during the week. You have to choose between the 80/20 rule and your cheat day.

How Does It Work?

This plan doesn't work by limiting your calorie intake, as lots of the more traditional 'diets' do. Look at our section on Diet Myths (pages 98–99) if you want to know why limiting calories is a really bad idea. Essentially our plan is a low-GI plan.

GI stands for Glycaemic Index, and refers to the score given to foods according to how quickly they release their sugar into the bloodstream. This system was first developed to help diabetics control their blood sugar levels, but it's a really useful and healthy way of eating for the rest of us too. Foods with a high GI score are those that convert quickly into glucose within the body. To deal with this surge in sugar levels, the body releases insulin, which helps your body's cells to use up the sugar. Doesn't sound too bad so far, except that when the insulin has, very efficiently, done its job, the resulting rapid drop in blood sugar levels triggers the brain to seek more: by making us hungry. And not only that, but insulin also switches muscle cells from burning fat to burning carbohydrates: not good news if you're desperate to use up that stored fat!

In contrast, when you eat foods that have a low GI value they release their sugar into the bloodstream at a much steadier rate, avoiding the surge in insulin and the subsequent hunger pangs as your body does its job. We're not going to ask you to worry too much about the specific GI values of individual foods. We've done all the hard work for you. Essentially, the foods on the Free Foods and Protein Foods lists are foods that are zero rated or very low rated, and the foods on the Healthy Options list are medium- and low-GI carbs that you can safely fill up on without sending your blood glucose levels soaring. If you're interested and want to learn more, there are plenty of books and websites that contain detailed listings of foods and their GI values.

We also recommend that for the first two weeks at least you try to cut out wheat and dairy. There are two reasons for this. First of all, cutting these two food groups out will automatically limit a lot of fattening foods, and second, some people are intolerant to wheat and/or dairy. An intolerance is different to a full blown allergy, which can cause an instant and potentially life-threatening reaction. If you're intolerant the food causes less dramatic but extremely uncomfortable symptoms such as constipation and/or diarrhoea, bloating, water retention with weight gain, itching and headaches.

Top GI Tips

Swap white rice for brown
Snack on fruit with nuts and seeds as the protein in the nuts will help to stabilize blood sugar levels
Don't miss meals – try to eat every three hours
Avoid processed foods and go for natural, fresh produce whenever you can

A Note About Comfort Eating

There's one reason, and one reason only, why this programme might fall. And that's you. Making you feel bad is not what we're about, so we're not telling you this so you can beat yourself up, we're telling you so you can do something about it. If you follow our rules there's no reason for you to feel hungry or deprived, so if you find it difficult to stick to the plan there's something else going on.

Lots of us eat for reasons other than hunger. These include:

- Stress
- Unhappiness
- Anxiety
- Anger
- Boredom
- Loneliness
- Frustration

These are habits that start for some of us very early in life, but like all habits they can be broken. If you find yourself tempted to eat when you're not hungry then:

1 Stop.

2 Ask yourself what you're feeling.

3 Ask yourself whether eating right now will make you feel better, or have the opposite effect and make you feel worse.

4 Go back to your diary and look again at your Personal Commitment and your goals. Is it worth jeopardizing all the progress you've made?

5 Call on a friend for help. Talking through how you're feeling could be just what you need. If there's nobody around right now then write it all down in your diary. Get it off your chest somehow.

6 If you're still feeling tempted, go back and repeat the visualisation on page 23. Tune in again to your personal movie.

Remember, the New You happened the moment you signed your Personal Commitment. You are not the same person that you were before so you don't need to behave in the same way.

Choose Your Food

Portion Size

Yes, we know some of them are called Free Foods, but that doesn't mean you can eat as much as you like. Eating too much is one of the things that made you unhappy with your weight in the first place, so from now on you're just going to be sensible. We don't mean you'll be looking in despair at a plate with just three peas and one slice of meat on it, but moderation is best in all things. A portion size should be about the size of the palm of a woman's hand. So, a palm-sized piece of tuna with a palm-sized serving of sweet potatoes and a palm-sized serving of veg. Doesn't sound so bad now, does it? Remember to eat slowly so you know when you're full.

Foods that are high in calcium (see page 91) are marked with a **C** on the lists.

Free Foods

Vegetables

Artichokes
Asparagus
Aubergine (eggplant)
Baby sweetcorn
Bamboo shoots
Bean sprouts
Beetroot
Broccoli **C**
Brussels sprouts
Butternut squash
Cabbage (all types)
Capers
Carrots
Cauliflower **C**
Celery
Chicory (endive)
Chillies
Courgettes (zucchini)
Cucumber
Curly kale **C**
Fennel
French beans
Garlic
Gherkins
Green beans
Leeks
Lettuce
Mangetout (snow peas)
Mushrooms
Mustard and cress
Onions
Passata (tomato sauce)

Peppers (bell peppers)
Pumpkin
Radishes
Runner beans
Savoy cabbage
Seaweed
Shallots
Spinach
Spring onions (scallions)
Sugar snap peas
Swede (rutabaga)
Tomatoes
Turnips
Vine leaves
Watercress **C**

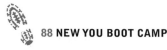

Fabulous Fruit

Apples
Apricots **C**
Bananas
Blackberries
Blackcurrants
Blueberries
Cherries
Clementines
Cranberries
Figs **C**
Grapefruit
Kiwi fruit
Lemons
Limes
Mandarins
Melon
Nectarines
Oranges
Passion fruit
Peaches
Pears
Pineapple
Plums
Pomegranates
Raspberries
Redcurrants
Rhubarb
Satsumas
Strawberries
Tangerines
Watermelon

Protein Foods

Meat and Poultry

Remove all skin and fat from poultry and all visible fat from meat before eating.

Bacon
Beef
Chicken
Duck
Ham
Pork
Turkey

Fish

Bass
Bream
Cod, plain or smoked
Dover sole
Haddock, plain or smoked
Hake
Halibut
Monkfish
Mullet
Plaice
Skate
Sole
Turbot
Tuna, canned

Oily Fish

Carp
Eel
Herring
Kippers
Mackerel, fresh or canned
Pilchards, canned **C**
Salmon, fresh or canned,
    plain or smoked
Sardines, canned **C**
Sardines, fresh **C**
Swordfish
Trout
Tuna, fresh

Shellfish

Clams
Cockles
Crab, canned
Crab, fresh
Crayfish
Lobster
Mussels
Octopus
Oysters
Prawns
Scallops
Scampi (but not
    in breadcrumbs)
Shrimps
Squid

Eggs

ALL eggs, either boiled,
poached or scrambled

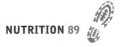

Beans, Peas and Lentils

Aduki beans
Baked beans in tomato sauce
Black beans
Black eye beans
Borlotti beans
Broad beans (fava beans)
Butter beans
Cannellini beans
Chickpeas (garbanzo beans) **C**
Garden peas
Lentils
Marrowfat peas
Mung beans
Mushy peas
Petits pois
Processed peas
Red kidney beans **C**

Nuts and Seeds

Nuts and seeds are fantastic, concentrated sources of nutrients, including omega oils, but are a high-fat option, so one portion should be no more than a tablespoonful, and you shouldn't eat more than two to three portions per day. You should opt for the unsalted varieties.

Almonds **C**
Brazil nuts **C**
Cashew nuts
Hazelnuts
Macadamia nuts
Peanuts
Pecans
Walnuts **C**

Hemp seeds
Linseeds
Pumpkin seeds
Sunflower seeds
Sesame seeds **C**

Milk Substitutes **C**

Calcium-enriched rice milk
Sheep's milk and cheese
Unsweetened calcium-
    enriched soya milk
Unsweetened soya yogurt
Whole goat's milk and cheese

Soya **C**

Soya beans (Not soy sauce,
    unless it's wheat-free)
Soya cheese
Soya flour
Soya yogurt
Tempeh
Textured vegetable protein
    (TVP) (textured
    soy protein)
Tofu, plain or
    naturally smoked

Some studies have suggested that soya protein may slightly increase your metabolism and encourage weight loss from the middle. However, as eating too much soya might also contribute towards hormonal imbalances we recommend that you only eat it in moderation, and not at all if you suffer from an underactive thyroid.

Healthy Options

● ● ● ● ● ● ●

In addition to your Free Foods and one Protein Food at each meal or snack, you can choose two healthy options a day from our Healthy Options list.

These are all store cupboard staples that you can make into hundreds of gorgeous meals. They're all nutritious and should be cooked without fat.

New You Boot Camp Granola
    (see page 105)
DelUgo spaghetti made
    from chickpeas
Oatcakes
Oatibix (2 biscuits)
Orgran vegetable pasta: other
    types of wheat-free pasta
    are heavily processed so not
    necessarily the best option,
    but are still preferable to
    regular pasta
Quinoa
Rice (brown)
Rice cakes
Rye bread
Rye flour
Rolled oats
Spelt spaghetti
Sweet potatoes
Wheat-free noodles

Flavourings

Savoury
You can have a little bit of salt to taste, but don't overdo it. Ginger, cayenne pepper and chilli can help to stimulate thermogenesis (heat generated by the body), promote weight loss, and speed up the metabolism. They can also help to reduce your appetite. However, you should avoid hot spices if you suffer from IBS as they can exacerbate symptoms. You can also use fresh or dried herbs, wheat-free soy sauce, and Tabasco sauce to flavour your food.

Spices
Cinnamon, ginger, cayenne, cardamom and ginseng can also help to stimulate thermogenesis (heat generated by the body) and promote weight loss. Cinnamon also helps to stabilize blood sugar.

Sweet
Agave nectar
Vanilla
Xylitol (available from most health food shops and
   some supermarkets: one
   brand available is called
   Perfect Sweet)

Drinks

Remember to drink plenty of liquids: aim for 2–3 litres (3½–5 pints) per day: mineral water, tap water, herbal and green teas. Limit caffeinated drinks to two cups per day: this includes black tea as it can affect blood sugar levels. If you don't like plain water try adding slices of lemon, orange or lime, or even a strawberry to add a little flavour.

If you are a coffee addict and fancy something different, try coffee alternatives that are made from barley or chicory (there is a brand called Caro Extra available in the UK). Avoid decaffeinated tea and coffee as they contain harmful chemicals and are not a particularly healthy choice.

Don't drink loads of fruit juice as it contains a high level of sugar and will raise your blood sugar levels quickly. This results in a slump that leaves you tired and in need of another sugar hit. One way of avoiding this is to dilute your fruit juices with water (about half water and half juice) and to eat something rich in protein at the same time.

Calcium

It's important for women to make sure they get enough calcium to reduce the risk of osteoporosis. If you're eating a dairy-free diet you can get your calcium from soya foods, calcium-enriched rice milk, sheep's yogurt, broccoli, cauliflower, kale, sesame seeds, sunflower seeds, almonds and tahini paste. Foods that are high in calcium are marked with a **C** on the lists. If you're still worried that you're not eating enough, you should see a nutritionist about taking a calcium supplement.

Potassium

Potassium-rich foods help to regulate both your metabolism and your body's water balance. Potassium is found in apricots, bananas, carrots, parsley, peas, spinach, salmon, sardines and cod.

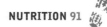

NEW YOU BOOT CAMP 10 COMMANDMENTS

Now you know the basics, follow our
10 Commandments to stay on track for success!

1 Never skip breakfast. This meal is essential to keep your metabolism working and give your body energy to burn. It's a good time to use your healthy option and choose a breakfast such as porridge and berries or scrambled egg and salmon on rye toast.

2 Drink plenty of water. A dehydrated body functions less efficiently and thirst can be mistaken for hunger. Aim for 2–3 litres (3½–5 pints) a day. Not only will you find your energy levels sky high, but also, as an added bonus, your skin will be glowing too.

3 Limit your caffeine. One or two caffeinated drinks a day is fine since it can boost energy and mental alertness. If you're used to drinking it, don't completely cut it out or your body will go into shock! Try fruit teas or red bush (rooibos) tea, which is widely available in supermarkets and health food stores.

4 Eat wheat and dairy free. We recommend that everyone should trial the wheat- and dairy-free diet for at least two weeks to feel the benefit. If you feel less bloated and have more energy and clearer skin, you can carry on for up to three months. Following an exclusion diet for three months should be enough to clear up any intolerance and you can then start to reintroduce wheat and dairy, but always in moderation to prevent the problem from recurring. If you still think you're having problems with wheat and dairy after three months, then it's worth seeing a nutritionist for some advice.

5 Don't skip meals. Going without food for too long allows blood sugar levels to dip. Eat three small meals a day and two snacks and make sure each meal has a balance of protein and carbs.

6 Eat slowly. Eat your food with awareness and chew it thoroughly to improve your digestion, so that you get more nourishment out of your food. If you eat more slowly you'll also find it easier to recognize when you're full and know when to stop eating.

7 Don't overeat. Large meals can drain your energy. Spread your food intake evenly over the day for constant blood sugar and insulin levels. You'll also find it easier to lose excess body fat if you eat this way.

8 Plan ahead. Stock up on some portable foods. The number one reason that diets fail is because people eat on the run or get hungry when there is no healthy food available. Keep your desk drawer, car or locker stocked up with healthy nuts and seeds and some foil pouches or ring pull cans of tuna, salmon or mackerel. Then whenever you can't get healthy food you've got something nutritious, filling and healthy that will sustain you all day and is a million times better than a sandwich and packet of crisps.

9 Be realistic – with your goals and with yourself. If you don't do this, you're setting yourself up to fail. Work around your own timetable. If you know you're not a morning person or have limited time in the morning, work out a suitable time to cook healthily, and stick to it! Preparing as much as possible the night before will help a lot here.

10 After the first two weeks, follow the 80/20 rule or have one cheat day a week. Perhaps you've followed diets in the past that revolve around sticking to the prescribed plan 100% of the time. The problem with this is that it's in our nature to veer off course after a while, usually out of frustration or boredom. Use our 80/20 rule and enjoy your life. When it's a friend's birthday, eat cake! But just have one piece. Once you're through the first two weeks you can celebrate special occasions with a glass of champagne or have a glass of red wine in the evening, just don't have the whole bottle.

Eating Fat

It might surprise you to hear that at New You Boot Camp we don't ask you to cut fat out of your diet altogether. If you want to lose weight it's true that you will have to restrict the amount of fat you eat, but in fact it's really important to eat a small amount, as long as it's the right sort.

Here's why:

- It can help increase metabolism
- It can help reduce inflammation
- It aids brain and nerve function
- It promotes healthy skin, hair and nails
- It can boost immunity
- It can help balance hormones
- It can help prevent heart attacks and strokes
- It transports fat-soluble vitamins A, D and E in your body

So, what is the right sort of fat?

☑ Essential Fatty Acids (EFAs)

Essential fatty acids (EFAs) are essential to life and can't be made in the body, so it's vital to eat enough of them. There are two main types of EFAs – omega 6 and omega 3. Most people eat enough omega 6, but it's harder to get enough omega 3, so it's important to include foods like oily fish,

nuts and seeds in your daily diet. While you're still trying to lose weight, however, you should remember that nuts and seeds are high in calories so you shouldn't eat more than two or three tablespoon-sized portions per day.

Olive oil is a monounsaturated fat, which helps to protect against heart disease. Like other oils, it should never be heated to the point where it begins to smoke.

Rapeseed oil is another oil that's relatively high in monounsaturated fat and it contains high levels of essential fatty acids too. It's also more stable at high temperatures than other vegetable oils, so is a healthy choice for cooking. Some of the oil that's sold as generic vegetable oil in supermarkets is rapeseed oil, and has the advantage of being much cheaper than olive oil, but do check the label carefully.

We recommend that you use no more than a teaspoon of olive or rapeseed oil for cooking or dressing your meals.

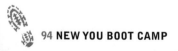

⊠ Saturated Fats

Saturated fat is bad for you because it increases cholesterol, which can block the arteries. Eating too much saturated fat is associated with obesity, heart disease, cancer and diabetes. It is found in foods like butter, red meat and full-fat cheese. You'll automatically exclude a lot of these foods if you follow our nutrition plan, but not all. Take care when you're eating meat to choose lean cuts and remove any visible fat.

⊠ Trans Fatty Acids

Trans Fatty Acids, or hydrogenated fats, occur when vegetable fats are processed or heated. If you follow our nutrition plan you won't be eating these anyway, but if you do eat processed foods or margarine, always check the label as these fats are even more dangerous for your health than saturated fats. If you're going to fry your food then use a teaspoonful of olive or rapeseed oil since these are stable at high temperatures.

Fat Rules   To make sure you get the right sort of fat:

- **EAT SMALL AMOUNTS OF SEEDS AND NUTS** – Mix one measure each of sesame, sunflower and pumpkin seeds, and three measures of a mixture of hemp and flax seeds. This mixture should be stored in the fridge in an airtight container – cold and away from the light to prevent deterioration. Add a tablespoon of these seeds to your breakfast each morning, or try them on salads or fruit. Grinding the mix in a coffee grinder helps your body to absorb the EFAs more efficiently, particularly for sesame, flax and linseeds. Use fresh seeds and nuts (unsalted) as snacks instead of biscuits and confectionery. Eat cereal bars made with nuts and seeds. Add nuts to porridge and muesli.

- **EAT OILY FISH** – A palm-sized serving of herring, mackerel, organic salmon, fresh tuna or sardines, twice a week, provides a good source of omega-3 fats.

- **USE COLD-PRESSED SEED OILS** – Ideally, an organic oil blend in a dark bottle, widely available from health food shops and some supermarkets. Use a teaspoonful at a time, cold, as a salad dressing or drizzled on vegetables.

- **ADOPT HEALTHY COOKING METHODS** – Avoid fried foods and try to steam food where possible. A small amount of cold-pressed, extra virgin olive oil or rapeseed oil can be used for gentle frying.

New You Boot Camp and Alcohol

You've probably always thought that it's all the calories in alcohol that are responsible for the way fat has a nasty tendency to accumulate around your middle if you drink too much. But studies show that on average less than 5% of the calories in alcoholic drinks are turned into fat.

The problem, when it comes to weight loss, is that alcohol reduces the amount of fat your body burns for energy.

When you drink alcohol, a small portion of the alcohol is converted into fat, but your body burns most of it off to get rid of the alcohol, using the energy produced along the way to fuel its cells and thereby dispensing with the need for your body to burn fat. For this reason we recommend that you don't drink at all during the two-week Drop-a-Dress-Size plan. Before you despair completely and throw the book away in disgust, once you've made it through the first two weeks, and as long as you follow a healthy eating programme and do lots of regular physical exercise, the odd tipple is permissible! Under the 80/20 rule, one glass of red wine with a meal up to four times per week won't do too much damage.

Red wine, especially Merlot, contains antioxidants that can help to protect you against heart disease and some types of cancer. There is also little doubt that TOTAL DEPRIVATION of anything

Top Tip

Remember the government guidelines for safe drinking state that men should drink no more than 21 units per week, with no more than 3–4 of these on any one day, and women no more than 14 units per week with no more than 2–3 of these on any one day. A pint of ordinary strength lager, bitter or cider or a 175ml glass of wine is 2 units, a pint of strong larger is 3 units and a single shot of spirits is 1 unit.

(food, drink, sex, love, fun, etc.) can lead to cravings and, ultimately, bingeing. We'd like you to stick to the odd glass, but we're realistic and we know that there'll be the odd night out when you just can't stop at a single glass, but remember, moderation is best in all things. If you find yourself falling off the wagon then follow our New You Boot Camp Drinking Rules to minimize the damage.

New You Boot Camp Drinking Rules

1 Remember, alcohol raises your blood sugar very quickly, so always have a protein-rich snack before or with a drink (a couple of oatcakes with nut butter, a small pot of live natural soya yogurt and a piece of fruit, a chicken leg, a cold boiled egg, some crunchy baby veg with a tablespoon of hummus).

2 For every drink you have, have a large glass of water (yes, you will have to go to the ladies room a lot, but you will seriously cut down on the amount of alcohol you have) and have a jug of water before bed to help rehydrate and ensure you feel great the next morning.

3 Remember, alcohol increases your appetite, lessens your resolve and removes those inhibitions, so try to make sure you have a buddy or partner around to keep you on track.

4 Avoid all fizzy mixers except soda water at all costs – they're full of sugar and even the 'diet' alternatives increase your desire for more of that 'sugar hit' and consequently more alcohol.

5 Avoid ALL 'lite' beers, 'alcopops' and 'ready mixed' cocktails – sugar, sugar, sugar!

6 Aim to drink only good quality wine or champagne (because you're worth it, darling!), or spirits 'on the rocks'.

7 Cocktails can be dangerously alcoholic and are often high in sugar, but if you stick to Martinis, Sours, Manhattans, Screwdrivers and Pimms (no sugar added, just the sweetness from the fruit), you shouldn't get into too much trouble. And, don't forget the highly nutritious, satisfying and delicious 'Bloody Mary' or 'Bloody Caesar', which surely have to be regarded as an essential part of any good, wholesome diet!

Dispelling Diet Myths

Surveys confirm what we already knew: that up to two-thirds of the UK population are unhappy with their body, with British women spending an average of six months a year counting calories. With such a huge audience it's not surprising that diet and media companies bombard us with advice. With conflicting voices on every side it can be difficult to sort out the useful advice from tomorrow's chip-wrapping, and dieting myths can soon spring up. So let's start dispelling them.

Myth Number 1
'Foods that say they are low fat are always the best option.'

It's true that most of the goodies that we crave are full of the saturated fat we should all be trying to avoid. So surely low-fat biscuits and low-fat ice cream must be a good thing? Unfortunately, things that seem too good to be true usually are. If you check out the ingredients you'll probably discover that they're packed with sugar and/or sugar substitutes.

You may be cutting out fat but you'll be wolfing down more sugars or sugar substitutes. Eating these products will cause a rapid rise in your blood sugar levels, which is why you get that feeling of instant energy afterwards. Your body responds by releasing large amounts of insulin, a hormone that helps your cells to use the sugar for energy. The bad news is that insulin is so efficient at getting sugar out of your bloodstream that it won't be long before you're feeling hungry, tired and moody as your blood sugar levels drop.

And if that isn't enough, while you're body is busy burning all that sugar for energy, there's no reason for it to start breaking down the fat that you were hoping to get rid of. So you'll find that you're not losing the weight you were expecting to either.

Myth Number 2
'I've been really good as I have only eaten one meal today!'

It might seem like a good idea to skip meals when you're trying to lose weight. Less food means less calories means less weight, right? It's not as simple as that. If you don't eat regularly, your blood sugar levels will plummet and you'll feel tired, hungry and irritable. It's much more difficult to resist the temptation of a sweet snack, or take the time to prepare a healthy meal when you feel like you have to eat, NOW.

On top of that, when you don't eat regularly, or you restrict your calorie intake too severely, your body simply switches into energy-saving mode: your metabolism slows down and you actually burn fewer calories than you were doing before you started dieting, making it harder to lose weight. This is a survival mechanism that evolved to help humans cope with periods of famine. When food becomes scarce your body naturally tries to hang onto as much of its fat as it can.

This is why we advise you to eat little and often. A good rule of thumb is every three hours. This will keep your blood sugar level steady, make you feel fuller for longer and give you energy throughout the day.

Myth Number 3
'All you have to do to lose weight is to eat less!'

Although we will be asking you to look at the size of your portions we won't be asking you to exist on starvation rations. If you go on a strict diet of 800–1000 calories a day, you'll lose weight at first. But, even if you manage to stick to such a strict regime, you'll quickly find that your rate of weight loss slows down.

This is because the survival mechanism we've already mentioned will kick in and your metabolism will slow down. Not only does this mean that it's harder to lose any weight, it's also the reason you'll gain back all the weight you lost, and probably a bit more as well, as soon as you start eating normally again.

The most effective way to lose weight and to maintain a healthy weight is to combine a healthy diet with regular exercise. That's why New You Boot Camp's two-week plan gets such brilliant results. It's not simply a diet plan, but combines a healthy eating programme with regular cardiovascular and muscle-building workouts. This combination of regular healthy meals and snacks with exercise will keep your metabolism high and ensure maximum weight loss.

New You Boot Camp Two-Week Menu Plan

Here we've given you a two-week eating plan that is perfect to kick-start your newfound way of healthy eating. If you follow this plan, your energy levels and mood will remain even throughout the day and you won't feel hungry.

If you follow the exercise plan in chapter two at the same time, you'll drop a dress size and feel full of energy. Our menus contain the perfect balance of carbohydrates, protein and fat to boost your metabolic rate and burn body fat. You'll find the recipes contained in the plan in the recipe section on pages 104–133. Once you've finished these two weeks, you can either carry on using our recipes and menu plans or be a bit more adventurous and try your own tasty combinations using the Four-Step Plan.

Week One

Monday

BREAKFAST: Scrambled Eggs on Rye Toast **HO**

MID-MORNING SNACK: 1 tbsp Mixed Seeds

LUNCH: Gomez Gazpacho with 1 tbsp Hummus and carrot sticks

MID-AFTERNOON SNACK: Celery sticks and 1 tsp peanut butter

DINNER: Red Lentil and Carrot Soup

Salmon Hoi-Sin (vegetarian option: Roasted Marinated Tofu) served with rice noodles **HO**

Tuesday

BREAKFAST: New You Boot Camp Granola **HO**

MID-MORNING SNACK: Butter Bean Spread with vegetable sticks

LUNCH: Cabbage, Tomato and Mushroom Frittata

MID-AFTERNOON SNACK: 1 tbsp Mixed Seeds

DINNER: Lentil Soup

Turkey Goulash (vegetarian option: veggie version of the Goulash recipe) served with brown rice **HO**

Wednesday

BREAKFAST: Scrambled Eggs and Beans

MID-MORNING SNACK: Cereal Bar **HO**

LUNCH: Salad Niçoise (vegetarian option: veggie version of the Salad Niçoise recipe)

MID-AFTERNOON SNACK: 1 apple and 1 tbsp nuts

DINNER: Mushroom Soup

Roast Chicken (vegetarian option: Spanish Omelette) **HO**

Thursday

BREAKFAST: Power Porridge **HO**

MID-MORNING SNACK: Cereal Bar **HO**

LUNCH: Chicken Cacciatore (vegetarian option: Rainbow Salad)

MID-AFTERNOON SNACK: Devilled Eggs

DINNER: Pea and Mint Soup

Sicilian Pork (vegetarian option: Veggie Bolognese and Courgette 'Spaghetti')

Friday

BREAKFAST: Scrambled Eggs on Rye Toast **HO**

MID-MORNING SNACK: Power Smoothie

LUNCH: Meatballs (vegetarian option: Seed Rounds)

MID-AFTERNOON SNACK: 1 tbsp Hummus with vegetable sticks

DINNER: Bean Soup

Mossaman Haddock served with brown rice (vegetarian option: Bean Burgers) **HO**

Saturday

BREAKFAST: Fruit and Yogurt with Mixed Seeds

MID-MORNING SNACK: Carrot Cake **HO**

LUNCH: Shepherd's Pie (vegetarian option: veggie version of the Shepherd's Pie recipe) **HO**

MID-AFTERNOON SNACK: 1 banana and a couple of nuts

DINNER: Tomato and Red Pepper Soup

Chicken and Ginger Stir Fry (vegetarian option: Vegetable Stew)

Sunday

BREAKFAST: Raspberry and Peach Smoothie

MID-MORNING SNACK: 2 oatcakes and 1 tbsp Hummus **HO**

LUNCH: Butternut Squash Soup with 1 chicken drumstick

MID-AFTERNOON SNACK: Dark Chocolate and Nuts

DINNER: Miso Soup

Thai Curry (vegetarian option: veggie version of the Thai Curry recipe) served with rice noodles **HO**

Recipes marked HO contain foods from the Healthy Options list and must be treated as one of your two healthy options for the day. You can swap these if you like as long as you don't exceed your allowance of two Healthy Options per day.

Week Two

Monday

BREAKFAST: Scrambled Eggs and Beans

MID-MORNING SNACK: 2 oatcakes with 1 tsp peanut butter **HO**

LUNCH: Crab Jambalaya (vegetarian option: Miso Soup)

MID-AFTERNOON SNACK: 1 tbsp Cinnamon Pumpkin Seeds

DINNER: Tasty Burgers served with salad (vegetarian option: Baked Falafel served with brown rice) **HO**

Tuesday

BREAKFAST: Power Porridge with blueberries and/or a banana **HO**

MID-MORNING SNACK: 1 tbsp Mixed Seeds

LUNCH: Tofu burgers served with salad

MID-AFTERNOON SNACK: Carrot Cake **HO**

DINNER: Spanish-style Chicken (vegetarian option: Vegetable Stew)

Wednesday

BREAKFAST: Berry Smoothie

MID-MORNING SNACK: Dark Chocolate and Nuts

LUNCH: Grilled Vegetable Open Sandwich **HO**

MID-AFTERNOON SNACK: 1 tbsp Butter Bean Spread and oatcakes **HO**

DINNER: Bolognaise and Courgette 'Spaghetti' (vegetarian option: veggie version of the Bolognese with Courgette 'Spaghetti' recipe)

Thursday

BREAKFAST: New You Boot Camp Granola **HO**

MID-MORNING SNACK: Chopped celery with 1 tsp peanut butter

LUNCH: Rainbow Salad

MID-AFTERNOON SNACK: Boiled egg

DINNER: Summer Vegetable and Baked Haddock Parcels served with brown rice (vegetarian option: Spanish Omelette) **HO**

Friday

BREAKFAST: New You Boot Camp Breakfast Smoothie **HO**

MID-MORNING SNACK: 1 tbsp Hummus and vegetable sticks

LUNCH: Asian Hot Pot (vegetarian option: Crispy Cauliflower served with Olives and Capers)

MID-AFTERNOON SNACK: 1 pear and a few brazil nuts

DINNER: Quick King Prawn Curry served with rice noodles (vegetarian option: Bean Burgers) **HO**

Saturday

BREAKFAST: Power Porridge with a banana **HO**

MID-MORNING SNACK: Soya yogurt with fruit

LUNCH: Butternut Squash Soup with Hummus and rice cakes **HO**

MID-AFTERNOON SNACK: Dark Chocolate and Nuts

DINNER: Pork Cutlets with Garden Vegetables (vegetarian alternative: Seed Rounds)

Sunday

BREAKFAST: Berry Smoothie

MID-MORNING SNACK: 1 apple and 1 tbsp nuts

LUNCH: Baked Sweet Potato with Roast Mediterranean Vegetables and Hummus **HO**

MID-AFTERNOON SNACK: Butter Bean Spread with vegetable sticks

DINNER: Thai Curry served with rice noodles (vegetarian option: Mediterranean Vegetable Medley served with brown rice) **HO**

Beware of Your Friends!

How many times have your friends said, 'Oh, go on, just this once won't hurt!' Sometimes they're right, and just want you to have some fun, and the New You Boot Camp programme allows you to join in and have fun when you need to. But if it's happening on a regular basis, you might need to ask yourself whether they have your best interests at heart, or whether they're feeling threatened by the new, more sorted, you. Just remember that you're in control. It's your body and you'll have to deal with the aftermath if things don't go according to plan, so don't be afraid to tell them that you're perfectly happy eating the way you are.

Recipes

We've only mentioned salt and pepper where a specific quantity is recommended; in all other recipes you're free to season to taste if you wish, but go easy on the salt! For fan ovens adjust the oven temperatures according to the manufacturer's instructions.

Recipes marked HO count as one of your Healthy Option choices. Some other recipes have suggestions for accompaniments that count as one of your Healthy Option choices. Don't forget, you're only allowed two of these each day.

Breakfast

Breakfast is the most important meal of the day. If you follow the old saying 'Breakfast like a king, lunch like a prince, dine like a pauper', you won't go far wrong. You need to kick-start your metabolism, get that body burning fat and set yourself up for the rest of the day, particularly if you're planning on doing some New You Boot Camp circuits!

Fruit and Yogurt with Mixed Seeds

Serves 1

2–3 tbsp plain soya yogurt
1 tbsp Mixed Seeds (see page 130)
2 pieces of fresh fruit, chopped

1 Put the yogurt into a bowl and sprinkle the seeds and fruit on top.

2 Serve immediately.

New You Boot Camp Granola

Serves 6

2 tbsp maple syrup
1½ tbsp molasses
30g (1½oz/½ cup) sunflower seeds
20g (¾oz/¼ cup) flaked almonds
200g (7oz/2 cups) rolled oats
1 vanilla pod (bean)

1 Preheat the oven to 150°C (300°F/gas mark 2).

2 In a small bowl, stir together the maple syrup and molasses.

3 Combine the dry ingredients and vanilla in a bowl, then pour the maple syrup mixture over and toss together.

4 Spread the mixture out on a baking tray.

5 Bake for about 15 minutes or until golden brown, stirring occasionally so the mixture browns evenly.

6 Serve with soya milk. Store in an airtight container for up to one month.

Scrambled Eggs and Beans

Serves 5

100g (3½oz/½ cup) dried haricot
   (navy) beans
1 tsp tamari
200ml (7fl oz/¾ cup) passata
¼ tsp xylitol
10 medium eggs, beaten
olive oil

1 Soak the beans in water for 8 hours or overnight. Drain, then simmer in plenty of fresh water for 1–1½ hours.

2 Drain the beans, then transfer them to a large fresh pan with the tamari, passata and xylitol and cook for about 15 minutes.

3 Pour the eggs into a hot, lightly oiled pan over a high heat and stir gently. Turn the heat down and keep stirring for 2 minutes or until the eggs are cooked and creamy.

4 Serve the scrambled eggs with the beans.

TIP: If you're short of time, substitute one tin of pre-cooked beans for the dried beans.

Scrambled Eggs on Rye Toast

Serves 1

2 medium eggs, beaten
olive oil
1 slice rye bread, lightly toasted
1 tomato, sliced

1 Pour the eggs into a hot, lightly oiled pan over a high heat and gently stir. Turn the heat down and keep stirring for 2 minutes or until the eggs are cooked and creamy.

2 Serve the scrambled eggs immediately on the rye toast with the tomato.

New You Boot Camp Breakfast Smoothie

Serves 6

600ml (1 pint/2$\frac{1}{2}$ cups) plain soya yogurt
250g (9oz/2 cups) frozen blackberries
    or blueberries
250g (9oz/2 cups) frozen raspberries
100g (3$\frac{1}{2}$oz/1 cup) rolled oats
1 tsp seeds
200ml (7fl oz/$\frac{3}{4}$ cup) apple juice
6 tsp agave nectar

1 Put the yogurt into a blender.

2 Add all the remaining ingredients and blend until smooth. Serve immediately.

Berry Smoothie

Serves 2

1 banana
600ml (1 pint/2$\frac{1}{2}$ cups) unsweetened/vanilla
    soya milk
100g (3$\frac{1}{2}$oz/1 cup) frozen strawberries
    or raspberries
1 tsp vanilla essence or almond extract
4 tsp xylitol

1 Peel the banana and cut it into large chunks.

2 Place in a plastic freezer bag, seal and freeze for at least 5–6 hours or overnight.

3 Take the banana out of the freezer and place with all the remaining ingredients in a blender or food processor. Blend until smooth and serve immediately.

Raspberry and Peach Smoothie

Serves 2

600ml (1 pint/2½ cups) unsweetened soya milk
250ml (9fl oz/1 cup) plain soya yogurt
150g (5oz/1 cup) frozen sliced peaches
75g (3oz/½ cup) frozen raspberries
1 tsp vanilla essence
½ tsp almond extract
fresh mint (optional)

1   Place all the ingredients in a blender and process until smooth.

2   Serve immediately in tall glasses. Garnish with fresh mint if desired.

Good food sources of omega 3

Hemp seeds

Oily fish (salmon, tuna, mackerel, herrings, sardines, pilchards)

Walnuts

Flax/Linseeds

Pumpkin seeds

Power Porridge

Serves 6

1½ litres (2½ pints/6¼ cups) water
300g (11oz/3 cups) jumbo oats
1 tsp ground cinnamon
3 apples
300ml (½ pint/1¼ cups) soya milk
2 tbsp sunflower seeds
1 tbsp pumpkin seeds

1   Bring the water to the boil in a medium-sized pan, then add the oats and cinnamon. Simmer for 5 minutes.

2   Chop the apples and put them in a separate pan. Add a little water and bring to the boil, then reduce the heat and simmer until tender.

3   Remove the oats from the heat and add the soya milk, stirring well.

4   Grind the seeds and stir them into the porridge.

5   Ladle the porridge into bowls and place the stewed apple on top of each. Serve immediately.

Soups

Soups are great for concentrated goodness on the go. They're perfect to take to work in place of the usual dreary sandwich. If you don't have a microwave at work, then take your yummy homemade lunch in a wide-necked flask to keep it piping hot. You can make a big batch at the start of the week and freeze some if you need to. We add silken tofu to lots of our soups as it's a great way to add protein to your meal.

Lentil Soup

Serves 6

100g (3½oz/½ cup) green lentils
1 tsp olive oil
1 onion, peeled and finely chopped
1 carrot, peeled and finely chopped
4 sticks celery, finely chopped
600ml (1 pint/2½ cups) water
2 tbsp fresh parsley, finely chopped
350g (12oz/1½ cups) silken tofu

1 Put the lentils in a bowl and cover with water. Leave to soak for 8 hours or overnight.

2 Heat the olive oil in a heavy non-stick pan and add the vegetables. Cook until softened.

3 Drain the lentils, then add to the pan with the fresh water. Bring to the boil, then reduce the heat and simmer for about 30 minutes or until the lentils are cooked.

4 Pour the soup into a food processor, add the parsley and tofu and blend until smooth.

Butternut Squash Soup

Serves 6

½ tbsp olive oil
2 onions, peeled and finely chopped
1cm (½in) cube fresh ginger, peeled and finely chopped
750g (1lb 10oz/4 cups) butternut squash, peeled and chopped
600ml (1 pint/2½ cups) water
600ml (1 pint/2½ cups) unsweetened rice milk
250g (9oz/1 cup) silken tofu

1 Heat the olive oil in a heavy non-stick pan and add the onion and ginger. Cook until soft.

2 Add the squash, water and rice milk, bring back to the boil and simmer for about 45 minutes until tender. Add the tofu and heat through.

3 Pour into a food processor and whiz until smooth.

Bean Soup

Serves 6

1 onion, peeled and finely chopped
1 tsp olive oil
2 x 240g (8oz) tins mixed beans
500ml (18fl oz/2 cups) passata
300ml (1/2 pint/1 1/4 cups) water
1 tsp paprika
1/2 aubergine (eggplant), chopped
1 fresh red chilli, deseeded and chopped
1 small bunch fresh chives, finely chopped

1   Sauté the onion in the olive oil
    until soft.

2   Add all the remaining ingredients except
    the chives and simmer for 15 minutes.

3   Pour the soup into a food processor,
    add the chives and blend well.

Pea and Mint Soup

Serves 6

2 onions, peeled and finely chopped
2 sticks celery, chopped
1 tsp olive oil
600ml (1 pint/2 1/2 cups) water
300g (11oz/2 cups) frozen peas
1 small bunch fresh mint, finely chopped

1   Sauté the onions and celery in the olive
    oil until soft. Add the water and bring
    to the boil.

2   Add the peas.

3   Simmer for about 5 minutes. Pour the
    soup into a food processor, add the mint
    and blend well.

Tomato and Red Pepper Soup

Serves 6

1 red (bell) pepper, deseeded and finely chopped
1 fresh red chilli, deseeded and finely chopped
2 sticks celery, finely chopped
1 onion, peeled and finely chopped
1 tsp olive oil
300ml (1/2 pint/1 1/4 cups) passata
125ml (4 1/2fl oz/1/2 cup) unsweetened rice milk
1 tsp paprika

1   Sauté the chopped pepper, chilli, celery
    and onion in the olive oil until soft.

2   Add the passata, rice milk and paprika
    and simmer for about 15 minutes.

3   Pour into a food processor and whiz
    until smooth.

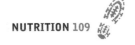

Miso Soup

Serves 6

600ml (1 pint/2¹/₂ cups) water
¹/₂ garlic clove, peeled and finely chopped
1cm (¹/₂in) cube fresh ginger, peeled and
   finely chopped
2 tbsp brown miso
200g (7oz/³/₄ cup) firm tofu, cut into small
   cubes
1 red (bell) pepper, deseeded and finely sliced
2 spring onions (scallions), finely sliced along
   the length
50g (2oz/¹/₄ cup) bean sprouts
1 small bunch fresh coriander (cilantro),
   finely chopped

1   Pour the water into a pan and bring
    to the boil. Add the garlic and ginger.

2   Turn the heat down and stir in the miso.
    Add the cubed tofu and heat through.

3   Divide the sliced pepper, spring onions,
    bean sprouts and coriander between
    your serving bowls, fish out the tofu
    from the broth and add to the bowls,
    then pour the soup over the top.

Gomez Gazpacho

Serves 4

5 ripe big juicy tomatoes, roughly chopped
1 cucumber, roughly chopped
1 red (bell) pepper, deseeded and
   roughly chopped
1 onion, peeled and roughly chopped
1–2 small garlic cloves, peeled and
   roughly chopped
2–3 tsp balsamic vinegar
1 tbsp olive oil

1   Place all the ingredients except
    the vinegar and olive oil in a food
    processor, add a splash of water and
    whiz until smooth.

2   Add the vinegar and olive oil
    and blend again.

3   Pour the gazpacho into a bowl and
    chill in the fridge for at least an hour.
    Serve cold. You may garnish with some
    Parma ham or a boiled egg, chopped
    and sprinkled on top.

TIP: If you prefer, you can skin the
tomatoes by scoring a cross in the top
with a knife, immersing them in boiling
water for 30 seconds and then removing
the skin with a sharp knife. You can
also skin the peppers by grilling them
until the skin starts to char, then
leaving them to cool slightly before
peeling the skin off.

Red Lentil and Carrot Soup

Serves 6

1 tbsp olive oil
1 onion, peeled and finely chopped
100g (3½oz/½ cup) red lentils
2 carrots, peeled and finely chopped
1 tsp ground cumin
1 tsp caraway seeds
1 litre (1¾ pints/4 cups) water
1 small bunch fresh coriander
   (cilantro), finely chopped

1   Heat the olive oil in a heavy non-stick
    pan and add the onion. Cook until soft.

2   Add all the remaining ingredients
    except the coriander.

3   Simmer for about 20 minutes until
    the lentils are soft, adding more water
    if necessary.

4   Transfer the soup to a food processor,
    add the coriander and blend.

Mushroom Soup

Serves 6

200g (7oz/2 cups) mushrooms, sliced
1 garlic clove, peeled and finely chopped
1 onion, peeled and finely chopped
1 tsp olive oil
110ml (4fl oz/½ cup) water
300ml (½ pint/1¼ cups) unsweetened
   rice milk
350g (12oz/1½ cups) silken tofu
2 tbsp fresh parsley, chopped

1   Sauté the mushrooms, garlic and onion
    in the olive oil until soft. Add the water
    and simmer for about 15 minutes.

2   Add the rice milk, tofu and parsley
    and bring to the boil.

3   Pour the soup into a food processor
    and blend until smooth.

Main Meals

These recipes can be used either for lunch or for dinner. Some of them can be made in advance and taken to work for lunch, while others are best cooked from fresh. Where a recipe lends itself to being served with one of your healthy options, we've mentioned this, but don't forget to count it as one of your two allowed helpings.

HO

Rainbow Salad

Serves 6

350g (12oz/4^1/2 cups) baby spinach
1 beetroot, cooked and grated
1 ripe avocado, stoned, peeled and cubed
1 carrot, peeled and grated
40g (1^1/2oz/^{1}/4 cup) cherry tomatoes
^{1}/4 yellow (bell) pepper, deseeded and chopped
125g (4^1/2oz/2 cups) alfalfa sprouts
1 tbsp chopped walnuts

For the dressing
2 tbsp olive oil
4 tsp balsamic vinegar
2 tsp agave nectar

1   Combine all the salad ingredients in a large bowl.

2   Whisk together the dressing ingredients and pour over the salad. Serve immediately.

Grilled Vegetable Open Sandwich

Serves 1

^{1}/2 small courgette (zucchini), sliced lengthways
^{1}/2 small red onion, peeled and thinly sliced
1 red (bell) pepper, deseeded and sliced
1 tbsp olive oil
^{1}/2 tsp fresh oregano
1 tbsp dairy-free pesto
2 slices rye bread, lightly toasted
2 x 50g (2oz) slices goat's cheese

1   Toss the vegetables in the olive oil and oregano. Arrange on a grill pan and grill under a medium heat for 2–3 minutes on each side until tender and slightly charred.

2   Spread the pesto onto the bread slices.

3   Layer the vegetables on the rye bread and put the cheese on top. Return to the grill for a further minute until the cheese is melted.

Spanish Omelette

Serves 3

1 tsp olive oil
1 medium onion, peeled and thinly sliced
275g (10oz/1½ cups) sweet potatoes, peeled
    and sliced
5 large eggs, beaten

1   Heat the olive oil in a medium-sized
    non-stick frying pan. Add the onion,
    cover the pan and cook until softened.
    Meanwhile, boil the potatoes for
    10 minutes or until tender.

2   Once cooked, drain the potatoes and
    add with the onions to the egg mix
    and stir thoroughly.

3   Put the frying pan back on the heat
    and turn the heat to medium.

4   Pour the egg mixture into the frying
    pan and turn the heat down to its
    lowest setting. Cook for a further
    20–25 minutes until there is virtually
    no liquid egg left on the surface of the
    omelette. Turn it over to cook the
    other side.

5   Cook for a further 2 minutes, turn the
    heat off and leave for 5 minutes to
    settle. Serve hot or cold.

Baked Falafel

Serves 5–6

2 tbsp olive oil
400g (14oz) tin chickpeas (garbanzo beans),
    drained and rinsed
1 small onion, peeled and finely chopped
2 garlic cloves, peeled and finely chopped
1 tbsp fresh parsley, chopped
2 tbsp chickpea (gram) flour
1 tsp ground coriander
1 tsp ground cumin
½ tsp baking powder

1   Preheat the oven to 180°C (350°F/gas
    mark 4). Drizzle the olive oil evenly in
    a shallow baking dish and put it in the
    oven to heat up.

2   Mash the chickpeas with a pestle and
    mortar or blend in a food processor.
    Add the onion and garlic and blend.

3   Add the remaining ingredients and
    blend to a thick paste-like consistency.

4   Shape into ping pong-sized balls
    and place in the preheated baking
    dish. Bake for 15–20 minutes, turning
    halfway through.

Quick King Prawn Curry

Serves 4

1 onion, peeled and finely sliced
1 tsp olive oil
1 tsp curry powder
1 tomato, chopped
450g (1lb/2 cups) raw king
    prawns (shrimp)
60ml (2½fl oz/¼ cup) water

1 Place the onion in a medium-sized pan and sauté in the olive oil until soft. Sprinkle with the curry powder.

2 Stir in the tomato and sauté for a few minutes. Add the prawns and stir to coat evenly.

3 Sauté for a few minutes until the prawns are cooked. Pour in the water, stir and bring to the boil, then serve immediately.

Cabbage, Tomato and Mushroom Frittata

Serves 6

1 tsp olive oil
200g (7oz/2 cups) cabbage, shredded
100g (3½oz/1½ cups) chestnut
    mushrooms, sliced
3 tomatoes, sliced
12 eggs, beaten
300g (11oz/4 cups) spinach
100g (3½oz/4 cups) watercress
100g (3½oz/1 cup) mangetout
    (snow peas), shredded
1 cucumber, sliced
3 spring onions (scallions), sliced
1 bunch fresh coriander (cilantro),
    finely chopped
1 tbsp tamari
juice of 1 lemon

1 Preheat the oven to 180°C (350°F/gas mark 4). Heat the olive oil in a non-stick ovenproof pan and sauté the cabbage and mushrooms over a high heat for a couple of minutes until tender. Drain well in a colander.

2 Cook the tomatoes in the same way.

3 Add the cooked vegetables to the eggs, pour the mixture into the hot pan and bake in the oven for about 30 minutes.

4 While the frittata is cooking, mix the spinach, watercress, mangetout, cucumber, spring onions and coriander. Whisk together the tamari and lemon juice to make a dressing and pour it over the salad.

5 Cut the frittata into slices and serve hot or cold with the salad.

Salad Niçoise

Serves 6

100g (3^1/$_2$oz/^{1}/$_2$ cup) green beans
juice of 1 lemon
1 tbsp olive oil
3 tbsp water
1^1/$_2$ cos lettuces, sliced
6 tomatoes, cut into chunks
1 cucumber, cut into chunks
2 tbsp black olives
3 x 200g (7oz) tins tuna
3 eggs, hard-boiled, peeled and halved
6 tsp sesame seeds

1 Put the beans in boiling water and cook for 2 minutes.

2 Whisk the lemon juice, oil and water to make the dressing.

3 Place the lettuce in a large serving bowl, add the tomatoes, cucumber, olives and beans and top with the tuna and eggs.

4 Toast the sesame seeds with a little salt in a dry frying pan. Grind.

5 Sprinkle the sesame seeds on the salad and add the dressing. Serve immediately.

VEGETARIAN OPTION: Use grilled tofu in place of tuna and add an extra egg. Crush a glove of garlic and mix with ^{1}/$_2$ tsp miso. Spread over the tofu before grilling.

Asian Hot Pot

Serves 3

450g (1lb) silverside or topside of beef (beef round), cut into stir-fry strips
^{1}/$_2$ tbsp olive oil
50g (2oz/^{1}/$_4$ cup) onion, peeled and finely sliced
1 garlic clove, peeled and crushed
75g (3oz/^{3}/$_4$ cup) pak choi, sliced or shredded
350ml (12fl oz/1^1/$_2$ cups) beef stock (broth)
60ml (2^1/$_2$fl oz/^{1}/$_4$ cup) tamari
^{1}/$_2$ tsp ground ginger
450g (1lb/2^1/$_2$ cups) broccoli, cooked

1 Sauté the meat in the olive oil until browned. Transfer to a slow cooker.

2 Add all the remaining ingredients except the broccoli. Cover and cook over a low heat for 10 hours.

3 Pour the meat and sauce into a heatproof casserole dish over a high heat and bring to the boil. Stir in the broccoli and serve.

HO

Shepherd's Pie

Serves 6

1 tsp olive oil, plus extra for mashing
2 onions, peeled and chopped
1 carrot, peeled and chopped
2 sticks celery, chopped
350g (12oz/2 cups) frozen peas
1 bunch fresh mint, finely chopped
1 small bunch fresh parsley, finely chopped
250g (9oz/1 cup) lean minced (ground) beef
250g (9oz/1 cup) minced (ground) chicken
300ml ($\frac{1}{2}$ pint/1$\frac{1}{4}$ cups) passata
1 tsp rice flour
250g (9oz/1$\frac{1}{2}$ cups) sweet potato, peeled
   and roughly chopped
300g (11oz/1$\frac{1}{4}$ cups) cauliflower,
   cut into florets

1 Heat the teaspoon of olive oil in a heavy non-stick pan and add the onions, carrot, celery and peas. Cook until softened.

2 Add the herbs, minced beef and chicken and stir until the meat is browned. Add the passata and a little water. Simmer for about 1 hour, stirring occasionally. Add the rice flour to thicken.

3 Boil the sweet potato and cauliflower until tender and drain well. Mash together with a little olive oil and set to one side.

4 Preheat the oven to 200°C (400°F/gas mark 6).

5 Put the beef and chicken mixture into an ovenproof dish and top with the mashed potatoes and cauliflower. Cook for about 15 minutes until golden brown.

Top Tip

Don't be tempted to skip meals if you're on the run. Choosing the healthiest option available is better than missing a meal, which will only make you more likely to give in to temptation later in the day.

VEGETARIAN OPTION: Replace the minced (ground) meat with textured vegetable (soy) protein.

Baked Sweet Potato with Roast Mediterranean Vegetables and Hummus

Serves 2

2 sweet potatoes
1 courgette (zucchini)
1 yellow (bell) pepper, deseeded
1 small aubergine (eggplant)
1 small red onion, peeled
handful of cherry tomatoes
2 tsp olive oil
Hummus (see recipe on page 130), to serve

1   Preheat the oven to 190°C (375°F/gas mark 5).

2   Pierce each potato to prevent them from splitting when baking. Place in the oven on a baking tray for around 45 minutes, or until soft.

3   Meanwhile, chop all the vegetables to roughly the same size as the cherry tomatoes. Spread out on a second baking tray and brush with the olive oil. Put them into the oven to roast alongside the potatoes for the last 20–30 minutes of the cooking time.

4   Once both the potatoes and vegetables are cooked, split the potatoes open and serve with the vegetables and a dollop of Hummus.

Turkey Goulash

Serves 6

1 tsp olive oil
2 onions, peeled and sliced
4 sticks celery, finely chopped
2 garlic cloves, peeled and finely chopped
4 tsp smoked paprika
6 x 175g (6oz) slices of turkey breast, each cut into 6 cubes
450ml (³/₄ pint/2 cups) passata
250g (9oz/1¹/₂ cup) green beans

1   Heat the olive oil in a heavy non-stick pan and cook the onions until tender.

2   Add the celery, garlic and paprika and sauté for 1 minute.

3   Add the turkey and stir to seal the meat, then pour in the passata and leave to simmer for about 45 minutes until the turkey is tender.

4   Blanch the beans for 2 minutes in boiling water.

5   Serve the goulash with the beans and, if you want to use one of your Healthy Options for the day, add some brown rice.

VEGETARIAN OPTION: Use grilled tofu instead of turkey. Crush a small clove of garlic and mix with ¹/₂ tsp miso. Spread on the tofu and grill until browned. Chop into chunks and add with the passata.

Thai Curry

Serves 6

6 x 100g (3^1/$_2$oz) chicken breasts,
    cut into chunks
2 sticks celery, finely sliced
^{1}/$_2$ leek, roughly sliced
50g (2oz/^{3}/$_4$ cup) mushrooms, finely sliced
1 onion, peeled and finely sliced
100g (3^1/$_2$oz/^{1}/$_2$ cup) Thai curry paste
400ml (14 floz/1^1/$_2$ cups) low-fat coconut milk
225g (8oz/3 cups) spinach
1 pak choi, sliced
50g (2oz/^{3}/$_4$ cup) baby sweetcorn
50g (2oz/^{3}/$_4$ cup) sugar snap peas

1   Put the chicken in a pan and dry
    fry for 10 minutes until the meat
    is cooked through.

2   Put the celery, leek, mushrooms, onion
    and Thai curry paste in a separate,
    heavy non-stick pan over a low heat
    and cook until they are tender.

3   Add the coconut milk and bring
    to the boil. Add the spinach.

4   Add the pak choi, sweetcorn and peas
    and warm through.

5   Divide the vegetables and chicken
    between serving bowls and serve
    immediately.

**VEGETARIAN OPTION: Cook this dish
with tofu instead of chicken, but make
sure you buy a Thai curry paste that
doesn't contain fish.**

Chicken and Ginger Stir Fry

Serves 4

100ml (3^1/$_2$fl oz/^{1}/$_3$ cup) chicken stock (broth)
1 tbsp tamari
1 tbsp cornflour (cornstarch)
^{1}/$_8$ tsp freshly ground black pepper
2 skinless, boneless chicken breasts, cut into
    1cm (^{1}/$_2$in) pieces
1 tbsp groundnut (peanut) oil
175g (6oz/1^1/$_4$ cups) mangetout (snow peas)
100g (3^1/$_2$oz/1 cup) mushrooms, sliced
1 green (bell) pepper, deseeded and finely sliced
2 tbsp spring onions (scallions), finely sliced
^{1}/$_4$ tsp finely chopped fresh ginger

1   In a shallow dish, combine the chicken
    stock, tamari, cornflour and pepper.

2   Add the chicken to the dish and put
    in the fridge for 1 hour.

3   When ready to cook, heat the
    groundnut oil in a large pan and add
    the mangetout, mushrooms, sliced
    pepper, onions and ginger and cook
    for about 5 minutes or until crisp.

4   Remove from the pan and set aside.
    Add the chicken and marinade to the
    pan and cook for 10 minutes or until
    the chicken is tender and the sauce has
    thickened. If needed, add a cup of water
    to the pan.

5   Return the vegetables to the pan. Cook,
    stirring frequently for about 2 minutes,
    then serve.

Women and girls who are pregnant, breastfeeding or who may become pregnant in the future should eat no more than two portions of oily fish per week. Women who won't have a baby in the future, and men, can eat up to four portions. This is because oily fish contains low levels of pollutants that can build up in the body over time and affect the development of a baby in the womb.

Bolognese and Courgette 'Spaghetti'

Serves 6

1 tsp olive oil
2 onions, peeled and finely diced
2 sticks celery, finely diced
1 carrot, peeled and finely diced
2 garlic cloves, peeled and crushed
1 tsp fresh thyme
1 tsp fresh oregano
1 tsp fresh parsley
1kg (2lb 2oz/4 cups) lean minced
    (ground) beef
500ml (18 floz/2¼ cups) passata

For the 'spaghetti'
6 courgettes (zucchini), cut into very fine slices
6 carrots, peeled and cut into very fine slices

1 Heat the olive oil in a heavy non-stick pan. Add the onions, celery, carrot, garlic and herbs and cook over a medium heat until the vegetables are tender.

2 Add the mince to the pan and stir until browned, then add the passata and bring to the boil.

3 Simmer over a low heat for about 1 hour.

4 Just before the bolognese is cooked, prepare the 'spaghetti' vegetables and cook in boiling water for 2 minutes. Serve as 'spaghetti' with the bolognese.

VEGETARIAN OPTION: Use 50g/2oz/ 1 cup per person of TVP in place of the minced beef.

Chicken Cacciatore

Serves 4

1 tbsp olive oil
1 chicken weighing about 1.5kg (3lb 4oz),
    skinned and cut into 8 pieces
1^1/$_2$ small onions, peeled and thinly sliced
2 large garlic cloves, peeled and finely chopped
2 tsp chopped fresh rosemary
125ml (4^1/$_2$fl oz/^{1}/$_2$ cup) dry white wine
^{3}/$_4$ tsp salt
^{1}/$_4$ tsp crushed chilli flakes
225g (8oz/1 cup) tinned plum tomatoes,
    drained, 1 coarsely chopped

1 In a large pan, heat the olive oil over a
   medium-high heat. Brown the chicken in
   two batches, cooking each batch for about
   8 minutes. Transfer to a plate.

2 Add the onion, garlic and rosemary to
   the pan and cook for about 4 minutes until
   the onion is soft. Add the wine and bring
   to a boil, stirring to loosen any browned
   bits. Add the salt and chilli flakes.

3 Return the chicken, and any juices from
   the plate, to the pan. Boil until almost
   all the wine has evaporated – about 2
   minutes. Add the tomatoes. Cover, reduce
   the heat to low and simmer for 30
   minutes until the chicken is
   cooked through.

4 Transfer the chicken to a serving plate.
   Boil the sauce for a further 2 minutes to
   thicken before spooning over the chicken
   and serving.

Crispy Cauliflower Served with Olives and Capers

Serves 6

50g (2oz/^{1}/$_4$ cup) black olives, finely chopped
2 tsp capers, drained and finely chopped
1 tbsp red wine vinegar
2 tbsp olive oil plus 1 tsp
1.8kg (4lb/7^1/$_2$ cups) cauliflower florets
2 tbsp fresh parsley, finely chopped
6 tbsp flaked almonds, toasted

1 Combine the olives, capers and vinegar
   with 2 tbsp of olive oil in a bowl.

2 Heat the remaining oil in a heavy non-
   stick pan over medium-high heat and
   cook the cauliflower for 10 minutes,
   covered, stirring occasionally.

3 Uncover the pan and sauté the
   cauliflower for another 5–10 minutes,
   until tender and browned.

4 Transfer the cauliflower to a bowl
   and toss with the olive mixture and the
   parsley. Serve with the flaked almonds
   sprinkled over the top.

TIP: Meat eaters can leave out the
almonds and serve this as a side dish
with any sort of protein, for example
baked chicken breasts or grilled
salmon steaks.

Spanish-style Chicken

Serves 4

6 chicken breasts, skinned and halved
1/4 tsp freshly ground black pepper
cooking oil spray
1 medium onion, peeled and finely sliced
1 garlic clove, peeled and finely chopped
200g (7oz/2 cups) mushrooms, sliced
240ml (8½fl oz/1 cup) water plus 2 tbsp water
2 tsp paprika
1 tsp dry chicken stock (bouillon) powder
½ tsp saffron threads (or turmeric)
240g (8½oz/1½ cups) frozen peas
2 tbsp olives, pitted and sliced
60ml (2½fl oz/¼ cup) unsweetened
    soya milk
1 tbsp cornflour (cornstarch)
700g (1½lb/3 cups) mixed green
    vegetables such as mangetout (snow peas),
    asparagus, green beans

1   Sprinkle the chicken with the pepper.
    Coat the interior of a large flameproof
    casserole dish with the cooking oil
    spray and place the chicken in. Cook
    over a medium heat until browned,
    then remove from the pan. Soak up
    most of the fat from the casserole
    dish with a paper towel. Place over
    a medium-high heat until hot.

2   Add the onion, garlic and mushrooms
    and sauté until tender. Add the chicken,
    1 cup of water, paprika, stock powder
    and saffron threads. Bring to a boil.
    Cover, reduce heat and simmer for
    25 minutes until the chicken is tender.
    Remove the chicken and set aside.

3   Add the peas, olives and soya milk to
    the casserole dish. Cover and simmer
    for 5 minutes. Combine the cornflour
    with the remaining 2 tbsp water and
    add to the sauce mixture. Bring to the
    boil. Reduce the heat and cook, stirring
    constantly until thickened and bubbly.
    Remove from the heat.

4   Blanch the green vegetable medley
    for 2–3 minutes. Drain well.

5   Serve the chicken on top of the green
    vegetables. Top with the sauce.

Summer Vegetable and Baked Haddock Parcels

Serves 4

1 tsp olive oil
450g (1lb) haddock fillets
$^1/_2$ red (bell) pepper, deseeded and sliced
2 courgettes (zucchini), sliced
8 shallots, peeled and halved
1 garlic clove, peeled and crushed

1   Preheat the oven to 230°C (450°F/ gas mark 8).

2   Coat the centre of 4 sheets of foil measuring 45 x 45cm (18 x18in) with a drop of olive oil and place one haddock fillet in the centre of each sheet.

3   Combine the remaining ingredients in a bowl. Divide the resulting mixture between the parcels on top of the fish.

4   For each foil packet, bring two opposite sides of the foil square up and over the fish and vegetables. Make a double fold to seal tightly. Fold the remaining ends up and over twice to seal tightly. Place the packets on a baking sheet. Bake for 20 minutes or until the fish flakes easily with a fork.

Vegetable Stew

Serves 2

2 tsp olive oil
1 medium onion, peeled and finely sliced
1 large garlic clove, peeled and crushed
250g (9oz/1 cup) butternut squash, peeled, deseeded and cut into 1cm ($^1/_2$in) cubes
1 red (bell) pepper, deseeded and chopped
2 courgettes (zucchini), diced
$^1/_2$ tsp ground cumin
$^1/_8$ tsp cayenne, or more to taste
$^1/_2$ tsp orange zest
400g (14oz/2 cups) tinned black beans, drained and rinsed
3 small tomatoes, diced
400ml (14fl oz/1$^3/_4$ cups) water
25g (1oz/$^1/_2$ cup) fresh coriander (cilantro), chopped

1   Heat the olive oil in a heavy non-stick pan over a medium-high heat.

2   Stir in the onion, garlic and squash. Stir in the chopped pepper, courgettes, spices and zest. Cook for 4–5 minutes, stirring occasionally, until the squash and peppers are tender.

3   Stir in the beans and tomatoes and cook for about 3 minutes, or until heated through. Add the water and simmer for 40 minutes until the vegetables are tender. Add the coriander to the stew just before serving.

Tasty Burgers

Serves 4

450g (1lb/2 cups) extra-lean minced
    (ground) beef
1 small onion, peeled and finely chopped
$1/2$ tsp freshly ground black pepper
4–8 tbsp sauerkraut, drained
1 tomato, sliced
4 thin slices goat's cheese

To serve
4 slices rye bread
4 tbsp egg- and dairy-free mayonnaise,
    such as mayola (optional)

1   Mix the beef, onion and pepper
    together and form four burgers of
    equal size, about 2cm ($3/4$in) thick.

2   Grill for 3 minutes on each side.

3   Place 1–2 tbsp of the sauerkraut and
    1 slice of tomato on the centre of each
    burger and top each with a slice of
    goat's cheese.

4   Grill for 2 minutes until the cheese
    melts. Serve each burger open-face on
    a slice of toasted or grilled light rye
    bread (this counts as one of your
    Healthy choices for the day). If desired,
    top each with 1 tbsp of the mayonnaise.

Crab Jambalaya

Serves 3

100g (31/2oz/$1/2$ cup) lean bacon, chopped
$1/2$ onion, peeled and finely sliced
50g (2oz/$1/4$ cup) celery, sliced
1 green (bell) pepper, deseeded and sliced
225g (8oz/1 cup) tinned tomatoes
1 tbsp Worcestershire sauce
350g (12oz/2 cups) crab meat

1   In a medium pan, fry the bacon until
    brown. Add the onion, celery and
    sliced pepper and cook until soft.

2   Add the tomatoes and Worcestershire
    sauce. Cover and simmer for
    10 minutes.

3   Add the crab and cook for 5 minutes
    until heated through.

4   Serve immediately. If you're using one
    of your Healthy Options, this is good
    served with brown rice.

Pork Cutlets with Garden Vegetables

Serves 4

2 tsp olive oil
4 pork cutlets
200g (7oz/1 cup) tomatoes,
   skinned and chopped
5 tbsp tomato purée (paste)
$1/2$ onion, peeled and finely sliced
2 tsp fresh chilli, deseeded and finely sliced
2 garlic cloves, peeled and crushed
juice of 1 lime
$1/8$ tsp ground cumin
175g (6oz/$1^{1}/4$ cups) carrots, peeled and
   thinly sliced
175g (6oz/1 cup) courgettes (zucchini),
   thinly sliced
$2^{1}/2$ tbsp raisins
$2^{1}/2$ tbsp almonds, finely chopped

1 Heat the olive oil in a heavy non-stick
   pan over a medium-high heat.

2 Sauté the cutlets for 2–3 minutes on
   each side until browned.

3 Stir in the tomatoes, purée, onion, chilli,
   garlic, lime juice and cumin. Cover and
   simmer for 20 minutes.

4 Add the carrots, courgettes and raisins
   and cook for a further 10 minutes or
   until the vegetables are tender.

5 Stir in the almonds and serve
   immediately.

Sicilian Pork

Serves 4

4 pork steaks (about 110g/4oz each)
2 tsp Italian herb seasoning
1 tsp olive oil
1 onion, peeled and finely sliced
200g (7oz/1 cup) chopped tomatoes
$1/2$ tsp ground cinnamon
1 tbsp honey
2 tbsp red wine vinegar

1 Season the meat with half the Italian
   herbs and add salt and pepper to taste.

2 Heat the olive oil in a heavy non-stick
   pan over a medium-high heat. Sauté the
   meat for 2–3 minutes until browned on
   the bottom.

3 Turn the meat over and stir in the
   onion and remaining Italian seasoning.
   Cook for 2 minutes, then stir in the
   remaining ingredients.

4 Bring to the boil, cover the pan and
   reduce the heat to medium-low. Cook
   for 6–8 minutes until the meat is cooked
   through. This is good served with
   brown rice and a salad.

Meatballs

Serves 6

100g (3½oz/½ cup) dried chickpeas
(garbanzo beans)
1 tsp olive oil
1 onion, peeled and finely chopped
2 garlic cloves, peeled and crushed
450g (1lb) chicken breast meat, chopped
2 tbsp fresh parsley, chopped
150g (5oz/½ cup) lean minced (ground) beef
300ml (½ pint/1¼ cups) passata
350g (12oz/1½ cups) silken tofu
9 spring onions (scallions)

1 Preheat the oven to 200°C (400°F/gas
   mark 6).

2 Put the chickpeas in a bowl, cover with
   water and leave to soak for at least
   8 hours or overnight.

3 Heat the olive oil in a heavy non-stick
   pan and sauté the onion and
   1 clove of garlic.

4 Drain the chickpeas, then blend with
   the chicken and half the parsley in a
   blender or food processor. Combine
   with the mince and cooked onion
   and roll the mixture into six balls
   for each person.

5 Heat the passata in a saucepan with the
   remaining parsley and garlic. Mash the
   tofu and add to the sauce to thicken it.

6 Cook the meatballs in a covered dish
   in the oven for 20 minutes.

7 Blanch the spring onions and serve
   with the meatballs and a little sauce.

Mediterranean Vegetable Medley

Serves 4

8 cherry tomatoes
1 aubergine (eggplant), diced
1 red onion, peeled and sliced
1 courgette (zucchini), diced
1 red (bell) pepper, deseeded and cut into 5mm
   (¼in) strips
2 garlic cloves, peeled and crushed
4 tsp olive oil
350g (12oz/1½ cups) roasted marinated
   tofu (see page 126)

1 Preheat the oven to 180°C (350°F/
   gas mark 4). Toss all the ingredients
   except the tofu together in a mixing
   bowl with a small drizzle of olive oil.

2 Spread the mixture evenly across a
   baking tray and bake for 25 minutes.
   Add the tofu and return to the oven
   for a further 10 minutes or until the
   vegetables are tender.

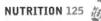

Salmon Hoi-Sin

Serves 6

6 salmon fillets, skinned and boned
1 tbsp hoi-sin sauce
200g (7oz/2 cups) bean sprouts
100g (3½oz/1 cup) cabbage, shredded
1 onion, peeled and finely sliced
1 yellow (bell) pepper, deseeded and sliced
1 carrot, peeled and finely sliced
1 tbsp olive oil
1 red chilli, deseeded and finely sliced
1 garlic clove, peeled and finely sliced
1cm (½in) fresh ginger, peeled and finely sliced

1   Preheat the oven to 200°C (400°F/gas mark 6).

2   Rub the salmon with hoi-sin sauce. Wrap the salmon in foil, sprinkle with a little water and bake for 10–20 minutes.

3   Put all the vegetables in a large non-stick pan (or wok) with the olive oil and stir fry with the chilli, garlic and ginger for 2 minutes.

4   Serve the fish with the vegetables.

5   If you want to use one of your Healthy Options for the day, this dish is good served with rice noodles cooked according to packet instructions .

VEGETARIAN OPTION: Replace the salmon with Roasted Marinated Tofu. Marinate 600g (1lb 6oz/2½ cups) of diced firm tofu with 4 tbsp of tamari and 4 tbsp of mirin for 15 minutes, then roast in a moderate oven for 10 minutes. Serve with a spoonful of hoi-sin sauce and the vegetables as above.

Seed Rounds

Serves 5

200g (7oz/1 cup) dried chickpeas
  (garbanzo beans)
1 tsp olive oil, plus extra for brushing
1 onion, peeled and finely chopped
200g (7oz/1 cup) textured vegetable
  (soy) protein (TVP)
1 egg white
1 tbsp fresh parsley, chopped
20g (³/₄oz/¹/₄ cup) ground sunflower seeds
20g (³/₄oz/¹/₄ cup) ground sesame seeds
20g (³/₄oz/¹/₄ cup) ground pumpkin seeds

1   Put the chickpeas in a bowl, cover
    with water and leave to soak for at
    least 8 hours or overnight.

2   Preheat the oven to 180°C (350°F/
    gas mark 4).

3   Heat the olive oil in a heavy non-stick
    pan and sauté the onion and TVP.

4   Drain the chickpeas, then put into a
    food processor and blend until smooth.
    Add the egg, parsley, seeds, onion and
    TVP and mix well. Add water if the
    mixture is too dry.

5   Form the mixture into 5 rounds, brush
    with a little oil and bake for 15 minutes
    until browned slightly. Serve with a
    simple tomato sauce.

Mossaman Haddock

Serves 6

¹/₂ tsp Thai red paste
¹/₄ tsp almond butter
3 tbsp coconut milk
100ml (3¹/₂fl oz/¹/₃ cup) rice milk
1 tbsp chopped fresh coriander (cilantro)
1 medium leek, cut into strips
1 red (bell) pepper, deseeded and
  cut into strips
75g (3oz/1 cup) spinach
6 x 175g (6oz) haddock fillets

1   Preheat the oven to 180°C (350°F/
    gas mark 4).

2   Fry the Thai red paste with the
    almond butter for a few seconds. Add
    the coconut milk and rice milk and
    bring to the boil. Turn the heat down
    to medium and add the coriander.

3   Blanch the leek, pepper strips and
    spinach in boiling water for 2 minutes,
    then transfer to a baking dish.

4   Lay the haddock fillets on top of the
    vegetables in the dish then pour the
    sauce over. Cover the dish with foil
    and bake in the oven for 15 minutes or
    until the fish is opaque and beginning
    to flake.

5   If you want to use one of your Healthy
    Options for the day, this dish is good
    served with brown rice.

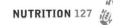

Bean Burgers

Serves 4

400g (14oz/2 cups) tin mixed beans
150g (5oz/³/4 cup) textured vegetable
    (soy) protein
¹/2 small sweet potato, peeled, chopped,
    boiled and mashed
1 tbsp fresh parsley, finely chopped
1 tbsp fresh coriander, finely chopped
¹/2 tsp smoked paprika
4 tsp olive oil

1   Crush half the beans, leaving the rest
     whole. Mix in all the remaining
     ingredients except the olive oil and
     form into four burgers. Chill in the
     fridge for 20 minutes.

2   Preheat the oven to 200°C (400°F/gas
     mark 6).

3   Heat the olive oil in a heavy non-stick
     pan, then fry the burgers for 3 minutes
     on each side.

4   Place the burgers on a lightly greased
     baking tray and cook in the oven for 10
     minutes.

Roast Chicken

Serves 6

2 tsp wholegrain mustard
1 tsp honey
6 skinless, boneless chicken breasts, cut in half
600g (1lb 6oz/2¹/2 cups) cauliflower, cut
    into florets
600g (1lb 6oz/3¹/2 cups) sweet potato
1 tsp olive oil, plus extra for mashing
400g (14oz/4 cups) cabbage, finely sliced
2 onions, peeled and finely chopped

1   Preheat the oven to 200°C (400°F/gas
     mark 6).

2   Mix together the mustard and honey
     and rub over the chicken breasts.
     Cover in foil and cook in the oven for
     20 minutes. Keep the juices from the
     meat.

3   In a large pan, boil the cauliflower
     and sweet potato until tender.

4   Drain well and mash with a little olive
     oil and salt and pepper.

5   Heat 1 tsp olive oil in a heavy non-stick
     pan. Add the cabbage and onions and
     cook until tender.

6   Serve the chicken, mash and cabbage
     with a spoonful of juices from the
     roasting dish.

Tofu Burgers

Serves 4

350g (12oz/1¹/₂ cups) firm tofu, mashed
2 tbsp tamari
1 carrot, peeled and grated (shredded)
2 garlic cloves, peeled and crushed
100g (3¹/₂oz/¹/₂ cup) textured vegetable
   (soy) protein
1 egg white
1 tbsp tomato purée (paste)
4 tsp olive oil

1 Mix together all the ingredients except the olive oil in a bowl.

2 Form the mixture into four burgers.

3 Brush the burgers with the olive oil and grill for 15 minutes under a medium heat, turning frequently.

Snacks

Two snacks a day are an essential part of the weight-loss programme at New You Boot Camp. Snacking between meals keeps your blood sugar even and your metabolism firing on all cylinders. That doesn't mean you can reach for the biscuit tin every five minutes! Here are some delicious and healthy snacks you can prepare in advance and keep on hand ready for when hunger strikes.

Power Smoothie

Serves 6

2 bananas
350g (12oz/1¹/₂ cups) silken tofu
1 litre (1³/₄ pints/4 cups) unsweetened soya milk
1 tbsp ground linseeds
2 tsp xylitol

1 Put all the ingredients into a food processor and whiz until smooth.

2 Serve immediately.

Butter Bean Spread

Serves 6

400g (14oz/2 cups) tin butter beans,
    drained and rinsed
6–8 sun-dried tomatoes
fresh coriander (cilantro), finely chopped
2 garlic cloves, peeled and finely chopped
3 tbsp olive oil

1   Put all the ingredients into a food
    processor and blend until smooth.
    Can be stored in an airtight container
    in the fridge for up to four days.

Hummus

Serves 6

400g (14oz/2 cups) tin chickpeas
    (garbanzo beans), drained and rinsed
2 large garlic cloves, peeled and crushed
juice of 1 lemon
1 tbsp tahini paste
2 tbsp olive oil
$^{1}/_{2}$ tsp salt

1   Put all the ingredients into a food
    processor and whiz until smooth.
    Can be stored in an airtight container
    in the fridge for up to four days.

Mixed Seeds

Makes 6 portions

50g (2oz/$^{1}/_{2}$ cup) sunflower seeds
50g (2oz/$^{1}/_{2}$ cup) pumpkin seeds
2 tsp tamari

1   Spread the seeds evenly on
    a baking tray.

2   Sprinkle with the tamari and stir
    well until the seeds are covered.

3   Toast under a medium grill for a couple
    of minutes, turning them occasionally,
    until the seeds are completely dry and
    browned. Leave to cool. Store in an
    airtight container away from light for
    up to four days.

Cinnamon Pumpkin Seeds

Makes 10 portions

1 tbsp egg white
$^{1}/_{4}$ tsp salt
$^{1}/_{2}$ tsp cinnamon
250g (9oz/2 cups) pumpkin seeds

1   Preheat the oven to 180°C (350°F/
    gas mark 4).

2   Beat the egg white with a whisk until
    foamy. Add the rest of the ingredients
    and toss well. Cover a baking tray with
    greaseproof paper and spread the seeds
    evenly on the tray.

3   Bake for 13–15 minutes until the pumpkin
    seeds pop. Let them cool completely and
    store in an airtight container.

Cereal Bar

Makes 30 bars

75g (3oz/^{1}/$_2$ cup) dried peaches
75g (3oz/^{1}/$_2$ cup) dried apricots
75g (3oz/^{1}/$_2$ cup) dried pears
75g (3oz/^{1}/$_2$ cup) dried cranberries
125ml (4^1/$_2$fl oz/^{1}/$_2$ cup) water
1 tbsp honey
1 tbsp molasses
50g (2oz/^{2}/$_3$ cup) desiccated coconut
50g (2oz/^{1}/$_3$ cup) whole almonds
20g (^{3}/$_4$oz/^{1}/$_4$ cup) sunflower seeds
250g (9oz/2^1/$_2$ cups) rolled oats
100ml (3^1/$_2$fl oz/^{1}/$_3$ cup) olive oil
1 tsp mixed spices
1 tsp ground cinnamon

1 Preheat the oven to 180°C (350°F/ gas mark 4).

2 Line a Swiss (jelly) roll tin with greaseproof paper.

3 Place the dried fruit in a pan with the water over a low heat for about 5 minutes until softened.

4 Add the honey and molasses.

5 Place the nuts and seeds in a food processor and whiz until broken up. Set aside.

6 Put the dried fruit in a food processor and whiz to a paste.

7 Add the fruit to the nuts, then add all the remaining ingredients and mix well.

8 Press the mixture into the prepared tin and smooth with the back of a wet spoon.

9 Bake for 20–30 minutes. Remove from the tin and cut into 30 bars. Leave to cool. Can be stored in an airtight container for up to four days or frozen.

TIP: Try walnuts or pecans instead of almonds.

Dark Chocolate and Nuts

Serves 1

small handful of nuts (almonds are
  a good choice)
2 squares dark chocolate

1 Toast the nuts on a baking tray under
   a medium grill for a couple of minutes.

2 Serve with the chocolate.

Still sticking to the NYBC ways: lost 23lbs in total now! I am so pleased! I have done various diets and got into exercising in the past but ALWAYS slipped back down the slippery slope. I know I have said this before but the New You Boot Camp philosophy has changed my way of thinking and I am not going back!

Sarah – April, Back to Basics

Carrot Cake

Makes 10 portions

150ml (5fl oz/^{2}/$_3$ cup) olive oil
75g (3oz/^{1}/$_2$ cup) ground almonds
110g (4oz/1^1/$_4$ cups) rye flour
1 tbsp baking powder
1 tsp ground cinnamon
110g (4oz/^{1}/$_2$ cup) muscovado sugar
3 eggs, beaten
grated zest of 1 orange
75g (3oz/^{3}/$_4$ cup) walnuts, finely chopped
75g (3oz/^{1}/$_2$ cup) dried cranberries
175g (6oz/1 cup) carrots, peeled and grated
  (shredded)
2 apples, peeled and grated (shredded)

1 Preheat the oven to 150°C (300°F/
   gas mark 2).

2 Grease an 18cm (7in) cake tin and
   line with greaseproof paper.

3 Combine all the ingredients in
   a mixing bowl.

4 Transfer to the prepared tin and bake
   in the oven for 1 hour or until a skewer
   comes out clean.

Devilled Eggs

Serves 6

6 eggs
$\frac{1}{2}$ tsp paprika
1 tsp dairy-free mayonnaise (mayola)
$\frac{1}{4}$ tsp freshly ground black pepper
1 tbsp chopped fresh parsley

To serve
6 lettuce leaves

1 Boil the whole eggs until hard-boiled (about 8 minutes). Drain and leave to cool.

2 Remove the shell from the cooked eggs, cut them in half and scoop out the yolk.

3 Mix the hard-boiled egg yolks with the remaining ingredients in a bowl, then pack the mixture back into the cavity in the hard-boiled egg whites. Serve each portion on a lettuce leaf.

Other Snack Ideas

- Soya yogurt with seeds or fruit

- 1 pear and brazil nuts

- Rice cake and Hummus (using recipe on page 130)

- Hard-boiled egg

- Oatcakes and Butter Bean Spread (using recipe on page 130)

- Celery sticks and peanut butter

- 1 apple and nuts

- Vegetable sticks (celery or carrots) and Hummus (using recipe on page 130)

- Edamame beans

- Tahini

- Go Lower bars (www.golower.co.uk)

- Rye crispbread with yeast extract or miso spread

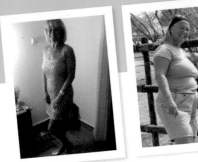

When I was younger I was very fit and active and so as I got older I never realized that the weight was creeping on. I'd never dieted in my life and it never crossed my mind that I should. Granted, I was finding it difficult to buy clothes that fitted and I'd noticed that shop assistants were ignoring me, clearly more aware than I was that nothing was going to fit. However, it wasn't until I was looking at some pictures of myself on holiday in India that I realized how big I'd got. By that stage I weighed 15st 7lbs and was wearing a size 18/20. I was horrified by the photos and knew I had to do something fast.

I wanted a tough regime and fast results, and I'd read about New You Boot Camp, so I booked myself in straightaway. In the month before I went I tried a crazy soup-only diet, which brought me down to 14st 7lbs. I thought that would make things easier when I got there, but I had a shock in store. I had no idea how unfit I was and struggled to run more that a couple of hundred yards. It was one of the most difficult weeks of my life. I cried a lot and was just grateful to make it to the end of the week. By that time I'd lost another half a stone and was determined to carry on the good work at home.

The New You Boot Camp fitness instructors gave me a programme to take home of running and strength exercises that I could fit easily into my life and I'd learned loads at camp about how to eat to keep my energy levels constant and avoid energy slumps that got me reaching for the wrong sort of snacks. More importantly they'd given me the drive and determination to carry on. As soon as I got home I booked myself on another New You Boot Camp to keep the momentum going.

A year and a half and three more New You Boot Camps later I now weigh 10st and wear a size 10, and it's all down to what I learned from Sunny and Jacqui. I run six miles every day now without even thinking about it and eat much more healthily. But what I love most about the new me is being able to shop for normal clothes again, knowing I'll look great.

I'm aiming to enter a triathlon soon, but not before I've been back to New You Boot Camp for the fifth time: not to lose weight this time but to help me reach my fitness goals.

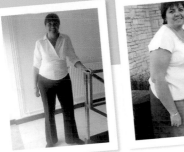
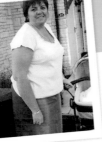

Before I booked on to New You Boot Camp my dad had just passed away. He was, and always will be, the most important man in my life, and I just started to pile on the pounds. I was getting more and more depressed and wasn't interested in going to the gym. All I wanted to do was to stay at home, and eat and feel sorry for myself. I was getting close to a breakdown and it just wasn't me. I knew Dad would be so angry and annoyed and I realized I had to start to do something. I'd read about New You Boot Camp, so I made the call. And I am so glad I did. What a fantastic week! I've never laughed, cried, worked so hard and been so knackered in one go before! I did things that I never thought I ever could or would do: abseiling, gorge walking, long walks, rolling around in sheep and horse... It's amazing what you do when you have to. Out in all weathers, we would all moan, but still would do it. The camaraderie and friendship that have come from New You Boot Camp are fab.

It was great as nobody knew who you were, or anything about you, and we were all there for the same reason: to improve our lifestyles.

And my God, have I! Since New You Boot Camp I have lost 4½st and have completely changed my whole outlook on life. Before, I would always put everyone else first and make sure they were alright – come New Year's Eve it would always be me on the phone ringing everyone. But not now. I am putting myself first for a change and doing what I want to, much to some people's annoyance. It's the first time for a very long while that I am feeling good about myself.

Hopefully, now I will find that special person too, as I have so much more confidence, and it's all down to my New You Boot Camp experience. I would definitely recommend it to anyone. It's the best thing I have ever done, and for me it has been totally life changing! Just wish my dad could see me now.

'I have lost 4½st and have completely changed my whole outlook on life'

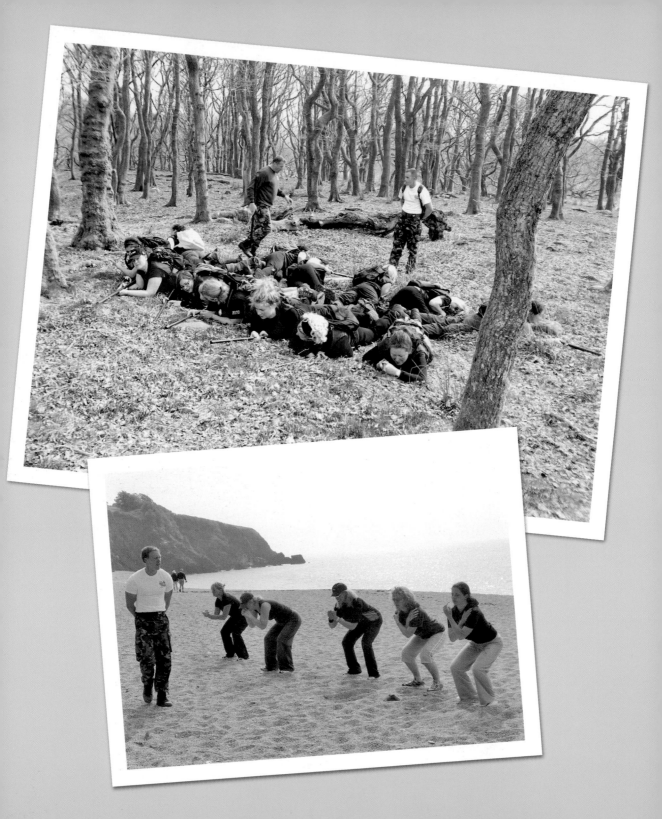

Life After New You Boot Camp

If you've followed the steps we've set out in our Nutrition and Training chapters you've come a long way towards making positive changes in your life, your health and your wellbeing. But we're sure that, like us, you've tried lots of diets before and know that it takes more than a two-week programme to deliver the permanent improvements you deserve. That's why we've taken a long hard look at what we can do to help you bring what you've learned from the New You Boot Camp programme into your everyday life. You've already got an eating plan that's flexible enough to follow for life and a set of workouts and circuits you can mix and match to suit your mood. What follows are some ways that you can apply those New You Boot Camp principles to different areas of your life so you can continue to feel the benefits for years to come.

New You Forever

This is the point where most diet and fitness programmes sign off. We've sweated with you through the training, we've shown you how to change your diet and we've cheered you on as you've achieved some amazing things. But unlike lots of others, we're not done yet.

Never Go Back

This is something we've been trying to emphasize throughout this book. You've made some important changes in your life since you started the New You Boot Camp programme, and we hope you've achieved your goals or are well on the way, but this is not just a programme that you can stop when the going gets tough. Even if you've reached your target weight, simply patting yourself on the back and forgetting about New You Boot Camp isn't an option. This has never been just about losing weight. New You Boot Camp is about living a healthier lifestyle that will keep you fit, your figure trim and your confidence brimming forever.

We know you're going to have the odd wobbly day – we all do! And because the New You Boot Camp programme is designed for real life it can cope with that. But what if your focus is waning and your wobbly days are starting to multiply? Don't just throw away all the hard work you've put in. Here are some suggestions to help you get back on track.

Look back at your personal commitment (see page 14). You made a promise to the most important person in your life: yourself! Don't go back on your word now.

Look at how far you've come. Have you added an 'after' photo, either on page 15 or in your New You Boot Camp diary? If not then now's the time to do it. You don't have to wait until you've reached your ultimate goal to congratulate yourself. Take a picture now and you'll see how far you've come. Look carefully at your 'before' photo. How did you look before you started the programme? How did you feel? Were you happy then? Are you happy to go back to living that way now?

- Revisit our motivational techniques on pages 18–29.

- Visit our New You Boot Camp Back Up Forum (see page 154). You can chat online with other people who are going through the same experience as you and share your problems. Check out some of the success stories on our website too and see how other people manage to keep their healthy lifestyles going.

- Shake up your routine. Have you started to feel as though you're in a bit of a rut with your training and meals? Why don't you try something different? Find some new routes to run, get out your bike or try a new sport altogether. Look through your cookbooks and find some tasty new meals you can cook while still staying within the rules.

Moving On

If you've managed to stay on track, then don't underestimate what you've managed to do. You've stuck to the New You Boot Camp programme with nobody dragging you out of bed, putting you through your paces or presenting you with your meals. That takes true self-discipline. You might have reached the goals that you set at the beginning of the programme or perhaps you feel you need to revisit those goals? We'd like to think you realize now that you're capable of more than you ever imagined, so if you've achieved one set of goals and want to set some more, or feel like you can stretch yourself further than you thought when you started, then now's a good time to review your goals

Start by re-reading Setting Goals on pages 18–19 to remind yourself how to set effective and achievable goals.

Think about where you might like to go from here. Perhaps you want to lose more weight or get fitter. We hope you've realized by now that the sky's the limit. You might not have thought you were a particularly 'sporty' person, but if you want to run a marathon and you believe in yourself, then you will achieve it.

Remember, you can apply the principles you've learnt to any area of your life. Do you want to go for a promotion at work? Do you want to get involved with voluntary work? Do you want to find a new hobby, save for the holiday of a lifetime or revitalize a tired relationship? You can do any of these things if you put your mind to it.

JO ROBERTS

After a car accident 15 years ago Jo's confidence had been steadily decreasing. She suffered from panic attacks while driving and avoided motorways. New You Boot Camp helped her to rediscover her lost confidence:
'On my return I decided that I was going to do my Mountain Leader training with a view to having a career based outside, which is what I love. I also took motorway driving lessons and am able to visit my parents via the M4, having overcome my motorway fear.'

New You Everyday Exercise

By now you'll know that exercise lifts your mood and gives you energy. So if you've got a case of the Monday blues or have a day of stressful meetings ahead, here are some quick and easy exercises you can do at your desk to help perk you up when you're feeling down. These will work equally well if you're not in an office but want to give yourself a quick pick-me-up at home. They're really not a substitute for your regular workouts and at-home circuit training from Training (pages 32–81), but if this is the only way you're going to fit in any exercise then go for it. Ideally, you should use these moves in addition to your everyday workouts for extra brownie points and extra energy.

Tricep Chair Dips

Sit on the edge of your chair with your knees bent and hold on to the front of the seat with one hand on either side. Taking your weight on your arms, move your bottom forward so it's just in front of the chair. Lower your bottom towards the floor, bending your elbows to 90 degrees, then push up again.

Why not get the whole office involved? Here at the New You Boot Camp office we have a whiteboard with all our names on and a chart with three different exercises on it. We aim to do three sets of 10 of each exercise and we tick our names off the chart when we've completed our sets.

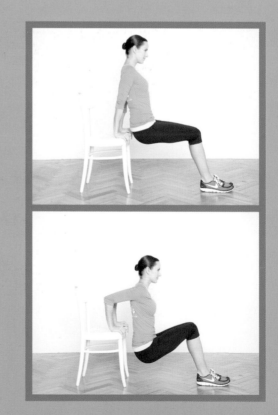

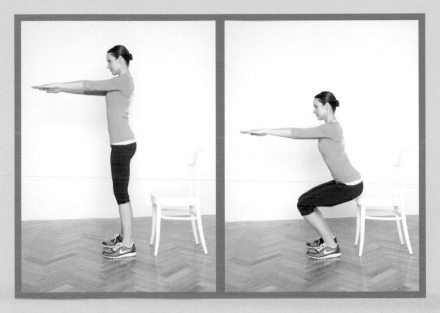

Stand Up, Sit Down

Stand slightly in front of your chair with your arms held out in front. Bend your knees as if you were going to sit down on the very edge of the seat. When your bottom touches the chair, push straight back up without putting your weight on the chair.

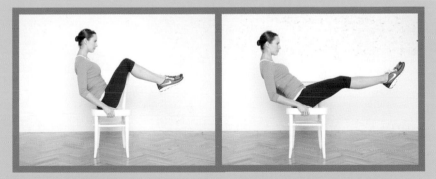

Roman Chair Sit Ups

Sit across your chair, leaning back slightly with your legs raised and knees bent to 90 degrees. Holding on to the seat, lean back and extend your legs out, then sit up again

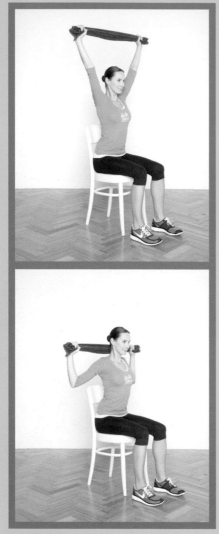

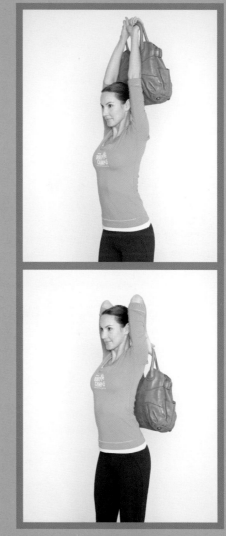

Towel Pull Downs

Sitting on your chair, take a towel or scarf and grip it at both ends. Raise your hands and the towel above your head. From there, pull the towel down behind your head, trying to pull the towel apart as you pull down.

Handbag Tricep Press

Sit on your chair with your arms extended overhead and your hands clasped around the handles of your handbag. Bending your arms at the elbow and making sure that the elbows do not move, lower your handbag behind your head and raise back up.

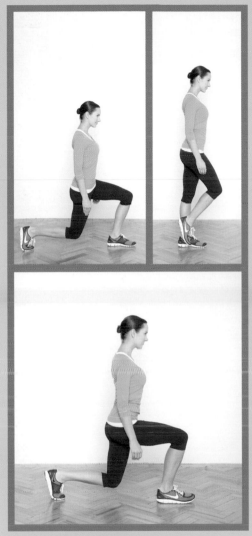

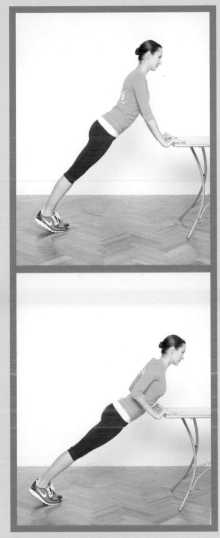

Walking Lunge

Stand upright with soft knees and your hands by your sides. Keeping your back straight, extend one leg forwards and go down into the lunge position. Raise up and step forwards and repeat for the other side.

Desk Press-Ups

Grip the side of your desk or table with both hands. Hold your body at a 45-degree angle to the floor. Lower your body gently down towards your desk until the elbows are just past 90 degrees, then push back up to your starting position.

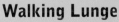

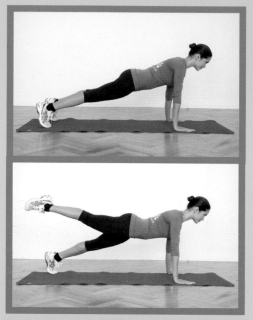

Prone Leg Lifts

Adopt the press-up position with arms straight. Hold the press-up position and raise a leg. Keep your leg straight and raise until it is parallel with the floor. Lower under control. Repeat using the other leg.

Top Tip

Pick an object like the photocopier that you walk to regularly. Every time you want to use the copier do the walking lunge there and back to your desk. If you're doing this at home you could lunge from the kitchen to the sitting room and back.

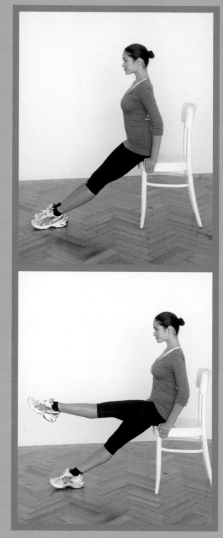

Leg Chops

Sit on the edge of your chair with both legs extended and heels on the floor. Raise one leg up until it is straight out in front of you, keeping the knee locked out. Gently lower until the leg is 15cm (6in) from the floor and raise back up. Repeat on the other side.

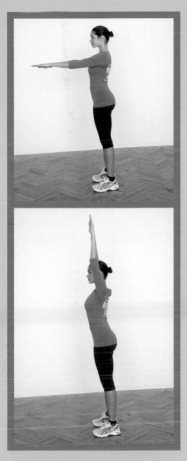

Arm Raises

Stand upright with your arms out in front at shoulder height, palms facing down. Raise your arms up to the vertical position and gently lower down again until your arms are parallel with the floor.

To add a degree of difficulty, hold a water bottle in each hand to increase resistance.

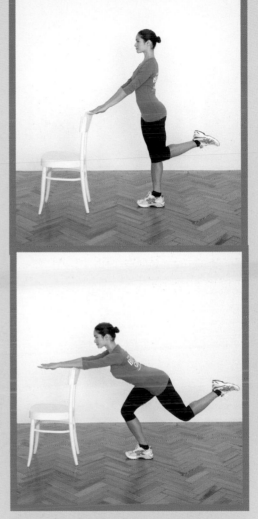

Single Leg Squats

Stand behind your chair facing forwards. Place both hands lightly on top of the back of the chair for support. Raise one leg, bending the knee to a 90-degree angle. Gently bend at the hip and knee with the standing leg and push back up, moving your hands forward over the back of the chair. Repeat with the other leg raised.

Get Your Family and Friends Active

A number one excuse that people wheel out for not getting enough exercise is lack of time. Most of us lead busy lives with careers, family, friends and domestic chores all jostling for a place in our crowded schedule. The obvious answer is to double up. Spending time with your friends and family and fitting in your training don't have to be mutually exclusive: take them along for the ride.

If you've got children we think this is not just a good idea but vital. Your children will copy your behaviour. Maybe not now, maybe not in five years' time, but in the long run, they will (don't we all turn into our parents?). By being active and showing your children how they can be active too you'll not just be giving them an immediate exercise fix (and getting your own), you'll be laying the foundations of a healthy lifestyle that will stand them in good stead for years to come. If you get this right then they'll never need to buy a book like this because a healthy lifestyle will be second nature to them.

So if you want your workout to be more of a social or family event, here are a few ideas to get you started:

● **WALKING**
This is the simplest and cheapest option. You can start out with no specialist equipment at all and it's suitable for even the tiniest member of your family. If you're short of time, it can be as simple as walking to the local shops whenever you can instead of driving to the supermarket. Take the opportunity to chat and point out interesting things along the way. If you've got more time to spare then why not strike out for the countryside with your friends? If you're going to tackle longer walks over rougher terrain then you will need to invest in some decent gear: proper walking boots, warm clothing, waterproofs, maps and a compass are all essential. If you've got very small children then a backpack-style carrier is a great way to get them

involved. If you're not sure where to go, look out for books or use the internet to find walks in your local area. If you're afraid you might get lost or just want to meet some like-minded people, look for guided walks or walking clubs.

CYCLING

This is another great social activity that children can join in too. It requires a bit more investment, as you'll all need bikes, but why not try hiring first? Check your local visitor attractions to see if they hire bikes out. Country parks are a good starting point and often have safe, car-free tracks that are a good place to start if you're a beginner or just a bit rusty. If your children are too small to ride their own bikes there are a number of options: trailers you can pull along, seats that fix to your bike or, as they get bigger, a bar you can use to tow their bike along behind your own. If you want to cycle on the roads there are several websites where you can check out safe cycle routes and cycle lanes in your local area.

ROCK CLIMBING

This is a good laugh to try with your friends or teenage children, although it goes without saying that it's not something you can have a go at without any instruction. Why don't you start by looking for a local climbing centre? They run courses tailored for beginners, often on indoor climbing walls, and will be able to hire out all the equipment you need. You can graduate on to rocks and cliffs as your confidence builds. There's nothing like the adrenaline rush you get from conquering a sheer rock face to make you feel there's no challenge you can't master.

SKIING

No, you don't have to splash out on a trip to Whistler or Chamonix. Indoor snow centres are the latest thing and are springing up all over the world. You can guarantee your children will love a skiing or snowboarding lesson, and you'll all get a wonderful workout too.

JOIN A TEAM

Whether it's netball, basketball, football or cricket, joining in a team sport is one way to make and cement friendships fast. It makes getting your training in seem like a piece of cake and whether you take a friend along or make some new ones when you get there it can give your social life a lift too. Look out for adverts in local listings magazines or use the internet to find a team near you.

OTHER IDEAS

Take your children ice skating or swimming or find out about sailing clubs or adventure holidays. Don't assume you're too old to start the same activities as your children. Lots of sports clubs have classes for adult beginners. Try a new martial art or why not give tap dancing a go? If you can get to London, book a New You Boot Camp fitness day for you and a friend.

What we're saying is don't rule anything out: having a go at new activities will keep you motivated and build your confidence.

Food for Special Occasions

The fab thing about our Four Steps to Freedom plan is that it's truly versatile. If you're eating out we'd like to think you'll find something you can eat and stay within the rules on pretty much any menu. See pages 150–151 for helpful hints on eating out.

If you're planning a special occasion at home, you're in control so you can stay within the rules, and we bet nobody will even realize that what they're eating will help them lose weight! We'd be proud to serve the recipes included in this book to any of our guests, or you can trawl through the cookbooks you have at home and you should find plenty of recipes that fall within the rules. Here are just a few ideas for different occasions to get you started.

Healthy Barbeque

Barbeques sometimes get a bad press, but are actually the perfect opportunity to eat healthily and well. The tastiest barbies consist of fresh, local ingredients rather than processed meats and white bread rolls. Find good-quality, locally sourced sausages and make your own burgers. You can serve these with healthy salads put together using fresh seasonal produce.

Stick to fresh fruit for dessert: juicy summer strawberries make the ideal sweet-tasting end to a meal. Try the smoothie recipe opposite for a fun summer treat.

Relaxed Family Supper

Menu 1
Main Course: Bolognese (see page 119) with Orgran vegetable pasta.
Dessert: Baked apples make a delicious and warming dessert. Core one large eating apple per person and stuff the middle with a mix of dried fruit and chopped nuts. Put the apples in a shallow baking dish with 4 tablespoons of water and bake at 200°C (400°F/gas mark 6) for 20–25 minutes.

Menu 2
Main Course: Meatballs (see page 125) with fresh, seasonal salad.
Dessert: Carrot Cake (see page 132) is bound to be a hit with all the family.

Menu 3
Main Course: Roast Chicken (see page 128).
Dessert: Take one banana per person, peel, cut in half and put them cut side up under a medium grill. Grill for a few minutes until the fruit is warmed through and beginning to soften. Transfer to a serving plate, drizzle with a little melted dark chocolate and scatter over a few toasted flaked almonds.

New You Boot Camp Summer Smoothies

We bet your guests won't realize there's no added sugar in this delicious recipe. Try it with other fruits such as raspberries, blackberries, mango and unsweetened cranberry juice as well. You can even take this with you to work if there's a fridge to store it in.

1 Peel and slice some soft bananas, hull and halve some strawberries and stick the slices in a tub in the freezer.

2 When you fancy a refreshing treat, and need cooling down get the frozen chunks of banana and strawberries and put them in a blender with either rice milk or soya milk or a little fresh orange juice (the less juice you have, the thicker the smoothie).

3 Add a teaspoon of flax seed, walnuts, almonds or pumpkin seeds to the mixture (this will help balance your blood sugar levels). Whiz the mixture in a blender and serve in long glasses.

Dinner Party

Menu 1

Starter: Melon and Parma ham. Opt for the best quality ingredients you can find and make sure the melon is ripe and juicy for the best flavour.
Main Course: Roast venison. Ask your butcher for a loin weighing about 750g (1lb 10oz) to serve 6 people. Sear the venison in a hot pan for 2–3 minutes on each side, then transfer it to a roasting tin and roast for 30–35 minutes at 190°C (375°F/gas mark 5). Take it out of the oven and leave it to rest for a few minutes before carving. Serve with roasted vegetables.
Dessert: Chocolate-dipped fruit. Choose dark chocolate with a high cocoa content.

Menu 2

Starter: Gomez Gazpacho (see page 110). Main Course: Salmon steaks topped with dairy-free pesto. Wrap the steaks loosely in foil and roast them in the oven at 200°C (400°F/gas mark 6) for 15–25 minutes. Roast some vine tomatoes alongside the salmon for a delicious accompaniment.
Dessert: Peel and chop 2 eating apples per person and put them in a heavy-based pan with a splash of water and 1 teaspoon of cinnamon. Cook, stirring until the apple breaks down to a purée. Layer the purée in glasses with New You Boot Camp Granola (see page 105) and soya yogurt.

Menu 3

Starter: Lightly steamed asparagus served with a poached egg.
Main Course: Thai Curry (see page 118) served with rice noodles.
Dessert: Take half a mango and quarter of a pineapple per person and cut them lengthways into thick slices. Brush with oil and grill for a few minutes each side until the fruit starts to brown. Arrange on serving plates with wedges of lime and fresh mint.

Golden Rules for Eating Out

We realize that if you have to travel and eat out frequently you might find it difficult to choose healthy food options.

It's easy to stick to the straight and narrow when you're cooking for yourself at home because you know what's in the food you eat. It's more difficult when you're eating away from home, but stick to our Golden Rules and you'll find you can enjoy a meal out without sabotaging your attempts to reach your goals.

1 Order a glass or jug of water as soon as you sit down. If there's something in your stomach, even if it is only water, you'll find it easier to control what you order and what you eat.

2 Avoid buffets. There's no portion control and the temptation to return for seconds is something you can really do without.

3 Trim as much visible fat and skin as possible from your meat before you eat it.

4 If there's a dish you particularly like, why not call ahead and ask for it?

5 Eat slowly, listen to your body and stop when you feel full.

6 Avoid gravies and creamy sauces. Don't be afraid to ask for a different sauce from another dish or for your dish to be served without the sauce.

7 Say no to the bread basket. Picking at bread before your food arrives will just add unnecessary calories to your meal.

8 Remember you're paying, so don't be afraid to ask for a different sauce or side dish.

9 You don't have to have the chips if they come as a side option – ask to swap the chips for extra vegetables or salad.

10 Try to order foods that are boiled, baked or poached and avoid anything fried.

11 If there's something you fancy that isn't within the rules, take advantage of the 80/20 rule. Life's too short to deprive yourself every time!

12 If you want to have dessert, you can stay within the rules by ordering fresh fruit or sorbet; avoid pastries and creamy desserts.

Food On The Go

A lot of ready-made food, such as sub rolls, bagels, cakes and pastries, contains wheat, dairy and the kind of carbs you should be trying to avoid. However, with a bit of inside knowledge there are a number of options to go for when you're out and about that won't do too much damage. Your meal should be based on salad or vegetables and a good-quality source of protein such as chicken, fish, eggs, red meat or nuts. The easiest way of achieving this is with a ready-made salad, tortilla, 'carb free' sandwich or wholesome soup.

The major supermarkets (including M&S) all have a good 'food on the go' selection. You should also look out for 'make your own salad' bars. Choose ready-made salads, antipasti and fresh soups such as:

- Spicy chickpea salad
- Mixed antipasti
- Tuna niçoise
- Classic side salad – add freshly cooked seafood to it or shredded chicken from the deli counter
- Edamame and butterbean salad
- Fresh soups

Fast Food Outlets

Most fast food places serve salads, but don't forget to hold the dressing.

If you're really stuck, fried chicken can be improved by removing the crispy crumb coating.

EAT Chain

They do a good variety of salads – avoid the noodles though.

Sandwich chains such as Pret a Manger offer a wide selection of salads and soups such as:

- Winter vegetable soup
- Carrot and coriander soup
- Chunky hummus salad
- Pole- and line-caught tuna niçoise salad
- No-bread falafel
- No-bread crayfish and avocado
- Super (duper) health and hummus salad
- Chef's Italian chicken salad

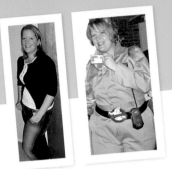

Josie Anson

I guess my journey started about four-and-half years ago when my twin sister asked me if she could borrow my clothes for a party. Normally it's not a problem – we often shared clothes in the past – except this time she was eight months pregnant and wanted to wear my normal clothes as her maternity clothes. It hit me quite hard when I realized I weighed over 14½st! I remember shopping for a party outfit and I had to get a size 22. I hated myself!

I joined Weight Watchers and lost a stone but couldn't keep the weight off. I threw myself into work but didn't resolve my issue with my weight or how I felt about me! I was really angry with my closest friends for not telling me how big I had got. In March this year my housemate sent me a mail with a link to the New You Boot Camp website saying, 'Fancy this?' To be honest I didn't even look, I just sent a message straight back saying, 'Sounds good!' Little did I know what I had just agreed to!

When Natalie and I arrived we all got weighed and measured. I weighed in at 13st

12lbs. That week was the hardest week of my life but also one of the best ones! I met some amazing people, who I am still in touch with. When you're halfway up a mountain and can't breathe it takes some pretty amazing friends and staff to make you realize you can get to the top!

At the end of the week we were re-weighed and measured. I was so nervous since everyone was having great results. I stood on the scales and the staff said, 'Oh my God, you've lost over a stone... well actually 16¾lbs!' I cried and so did they. It was official: I was the biggest loser and couldn't have been happier!

Back home I was determined to stay focused. Mum and dad contributed towards my planned holiday on condition that if I put the weight back on I had to return the money! I promised myself I wouldn't cash the cheque until I'd lost another 7lbs. A month later I weighed 12st 2lbs and banked the cheque! I got myself a trainer, who keeps me focused and works me hard once a week. He also weighs me, which keeps me on track. I now weigh 11st 11lbs and have just come back from the holiday in Antigua, where I felt fantastic in a bikini for the first time since I was a kid!

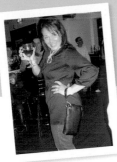
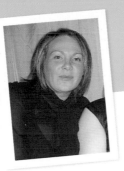
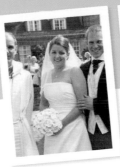
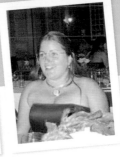

Sarah Bass

I didn't really tell anyone beforehand that I was going to New You Boot Camp but I've been telling everyone all about it since I've been back – even my clients! After I got back I went to a spa for the day. I got on the scales and discovered I was exactly a stone lighter than when I got to New You Boot Camp. I was in London so I went into Topshop on the way home and I got into a pair of Kate Moss jeans. How good did I feel!

I have continued with the diet and exercise and I have to say it truly has been a life-changing experience. I have now lost 2st, which I can't believe! You will be pleased to know that I haven't changed that much and still manage to have a few drinks (well, maybe more than a few) but, as you say, it's all about the 80/20 rule rather than the 50/50 I may have adopted before!

I know I have said it several times already but I can't thank you guys enough. I am soooooo pleased I went to New You Boot Camp, it has completely changed me.

Penny Rainbow

I was struggling to lose weight for my wedding day, so after reading up on boot camps and then researching on the internet for some time, I decided on New You Boot Camp. It not only kick-started me to carry on losing weight once I left, but also gave me the education to make life changes.

I have now changed jobs and am 16lbs lighter since I went to New You Boot Camp. I would like to thank not only the staff on my camp but also the team I have been in contact with since then. They have kept up the encouragement and helpful hints and tips. I can't thank New You Boot Camp enough for the New ME.

'I can't thank you guys enough. I am soooooo pleased I went to New You Boot Camp, it has completely changed me.'

New You Boot Camp Back Up Forum

Just as we hope you'll take the eating and exercise plans we've taught you here and carry them on in your everyday life, we'd also like you to feel that, even though you've come to the end of the book, our support and encouragement doesn't end here. We've set up a forum on our website where you can drop in and chat, to us and to each other, any time you feel like it.

Maybe you've got a question about something that's in the book? Or maybe you're just having a really tough day and need a bit of a boost. And don't forget to share the good times as well as the bad. We'd love to hear how you're getting on with the programme, and we know how inspirational your success stories can be to others in the same position. If you're doing really well, don't keep it to yourself: we'd all like to celebrate with you!

If following the programme in this book has got you wondering whether a New You Book Camp residential course might be for you, this is also the place to chat to people who've already taken the plunge and find out what it's really like.

To join in just log on to:

www.newyoubootcamp.com/forum

You'll need to register if you want to join in the discussion. If you have any problems you can contact us by email too:

enquiries@newyoubootcamp.com

"
I loved New You Boot Camp!!! I had a terrific experience and got out of it exactly what I wanted. I came back lean, toned and totally psyched to get back into regular training. It was exactly what I needed – a kick-start! Staff Woods was excellent. He was always smiling and full of buzz! He was sensitive to the needs of all of us and knew when someone was having a particularly rough day. At the same time he really knew his stuff and was always handing out little tips.
    Thanks again!

MARY DALLATT
"

Before getting to New You Boot Camp I had heard women say it had changed their lives, but part of me didn't really believe it. But after a week at camp, I'm a convert. Not only have I lost 5lbs, and 3 inches from my waist, my body has also totally changed. I have been this weight before, but have never had such a smooth silhouette, or been so toned. The difference really is dramatic. Now I can forget about dieting, and just concentrate on doing lots of fun exercise to maintain the weight loss. I feel like I can finally get on with my life and stop fretting about my weight and body shape. I'm so happy and grateful.

FLAVIA BERTOLINI

Hi there. Thank you so much for a fantastic week at New You Boot Camp, which I would highly recommend to anyone who wants quick results and a fantastic kick-start to a diet. What better way to go through torture than with 29 other like-minded, determined ladies. I couldn't believe the scales at the end of the week and I'm trying very, very hard to keep it all up. Good Luck with Portugal and, who knows, I may try to lose another 12lbs next year over there.

Three cheers for Staff Thom, Gough and Keast.

PAT BLACKER

I got back from New You Boot Camp early afternoon on Friday 25th September, having had the most rewarding week of my life. I managed to complete the week and tried everything and got great results. Not only did I lose 13lbs in the week, but my fitness level grew unbelievably. I went from just about being able to jog for 12 minutes to running continuously for one hour. I am not only physically stronger but also mentally more alert. The PTIs were fantastic and know just how to get the very best results: they spurred me on to do much more than I thought I could. The cold water barrels were surprisingly refreshing and very good for aches and pains. The week was tough without a doubt, but I have to admit I am kind of missing the place and the people now I'm back at home. I would recommend it to anyone who needs a kick up the backside, it's great to get you going. Thanks again!

DEB JONES

I am amazed that I have been able to do so much. It's a nice feeling. I haven't felt hungry and will definitely try to keep to the diet. I've met some lovely girls who really supported me during the activities. The New You Boot Camp has made a lasting impression on me.

Thanks so much!

JACKIE BULMER

Asian hot pot 115
bean burgers 128
berry smoothie 106
burgers, tasty (mince) 123
butter bean spread 130
carrot cake 132
cauliflower with olives
    and capers 120
cereal bar 131
chicken cacciatore 120
chicken and ginger stir
    fry 118
chicken, roast 128
chicken, Spanish-style 121
chocolate and nuts 132
cinnamon pumpkin seeds
    130
courgette 'spaghetti' 119
crab jambalaya 123
desserts 148, 149, 151
devilled eggs 133
falafel, baked 113
frittata 114
Gomez gazpacho 110
granola 105
haddock Mossaman 127
haddock and vegetable
    parcels 122
hummus 130
meatballs 125
mixed seeds 130
pork cutlets with garden
    vegetables 124
pork, Sicilian 124
power porridge 107
prawn curry 114
rainbow salad 112
salad Niçoise 115
salmon hoi-sin 126
scrambled eggs and
    beans 105

seed rounds 127
shellfish 89
shepherd's pie 116
smoothies 106, 107, 129,
    149
snacks 85, 87, 129–33
soups 108–11
Spanish omelette 113
summer smoothies 149
sweet potato 117
Thai curry 118
tofu burgers 129
tofu, roasted marinated
    126
turkey goulash 117
vegetable medley,
    Mediterranean 125
vegetable stew 122
venison 149

Roberts, Jo 139
rock climbing 147

self-assessment tests 13,
    40–3
skiing 147
sleep 14, 35
Smith, Vicky Ingram 93
sports clubs 147
success stories 30–1, 80–1,
    134–5, 152–3

team sports 147
Terry, Diana 11
time 9, 13, 36–7
Trainer, Helen 135

vision board 28
visualization 22–3, 28

walking 146–7

Ward, Tamara 80
water 14, 35, 91, 92, 97, 150
weight and BMI 40–1
weight loss 6–7, 8–9, 11, 28
    success story 30–1, 80–1,
    134–5, 152–3
weights 56, 57, 68, 69

Picture credits
Step by step exercise
photography by Caroline Molloy
(www.carolinemolloy.co.uk).
Models Tal and
Genevieve at Nevs.

Clothing kindly supplied
by Sweaty Betty
(www.sweatybetty.com)
and New You Boot Camp.

Author Acknowledgements

We would like to take this opportunity to say a huge thank you to everyone who has made this book possible.

Firstly we would like to say thank you to Staff Thom and Staff Lord, not only for all their expert advice and support on the boot camps but also for their input into the book and the training programmes. Alli Godbold, a big thank you to you for your nutritional input.

We would like to say a big thank you to all our clients for their ongoing support and recommendations and we do hope this book will help you continue on your paths to the New Yous that you have already begun.

Most importantly, we would like to say the biggest thank you to our phenomenal team at New You Boot Camp. Staff Balman, Staff Bishop, Staff Buckingham, Staff Cronin, Staff DeLong, Staff Evans, Staff Ferguson, Staff Ford, Staff Gough, Staff Keast, Staff Laskey, Staff Lord, Staff Rodder, Staff Straiton, Staff Thom, Staff Wheeler, Staff Woods and also to our fabulous boot camp managers, Kirstie and Pascale. Also, to all the team at New You Boot Camp Head Office for all of your support and hard work: Kelly, Lynsey, Danielle, Jan, Joanne, Diana, Austin and Nathan. All your loyalty and unprecedented expertise is a credit to New You Boot Camp and, without a doubt, is what makes us Europe's leading boot camp.

Finally, we would like to personally thank our friends and family for all your support and continuous belief in both of us and in New You Boot Camp.

Jacqui Cleaver & Sunny Moran

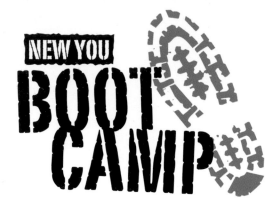

New You Boot Camp has recently been voted Europe's leading weight loss and fitness boot camp and one of the top military fitness boot camps in the world.

At our week-long residential boot camps in Devon, Somerset, Wales and Portugal, our team of world-class military trainers and highly qualified nutrition squad are here to help you reach your weight-loss and fitness goals. Our results speak for themselves, as do our success stories and testimonials. At New You Boot Camp we pride ourselves on making the difference in YOU that makes a difference in YOUR life. Our promise to YOU is that you will leave New You Boot Camp knowing that you can do and achieve anything if you put your mind to it!

We offer a wide array of different products that will suit all different clients with different fitness levels and different goals. We offer female boot camps, luxury and back to basics, male boot camps, mixed mid-week breaks and weekend booster breaks. We also offer New You Boot Camp military fitness days in London. Our most recent addition is the launch of our luxury retreat boot camp in Portugal, which offers both female only and mixed residential boot camps.

We are constantly introducing new products for our clients and it would be a pleasure to have you attend New You Boot Camp.

PLEASE TAKE A LOOK AT OUR WEBSITE

www.newyoubootcamp.com

OR CALL

0871 223 0066

31901050528860